The GP Training Handbook

Third Edition

EDITED BY

Michael Hall FRCGP

Institute of General Practice, University of Exeter,
School of Postgraduate Medicine and Health Sciences,
Exeter, UK

Declan Dwyer FRCGP

Thurlestone, Devon, UK

Tony Lewis FRCGP

Exmouth, Devon, UK

FOREWORD BY

Roger Neighbour

Blackwell
Science

© 1983, 1989, 1999 by
Blackwell Science Ltd
Editorial Offices:
Osney Mead, Oxford OX2 OEL
25 John Street, London WCIN 2BL
23 Ainslie Place, Edinburgh EH3 6AJ
350 Main Street, Malden
    MA 02148-5018, USA
54 University Street, Carlton
    Victoria 3053, Australia
10, rue Casimir Delavigne
    75006 Paris, France

Other Editorial Offices:
Blackwell Wissenschafts-Verlag GmbH
    Kurfürstendamm 57
    10707 Berlin, Germany

Blackwell Science KK
    MG Kodenmacho Building
    7–10 Kodenmacho Nihombashi
    Chuo-ku, Tokyo 104, Japan

The right of the Authors to be
identified as the Authors of this Work
has been asserted in accordance
with the Copyright, Designs and
Patents Act 1988.

First published 1983
Reprinted 1984
Second edition 1989
Reprinted 1990
Third edition 1999

Set by Graphicraft Limited, Hong Kong
Printed and bound in Great Britain by
MPG Books Ltd, Bodmin, Cornwall

The Blackwell Science logo is a
trade mark of Blackwell Science Ltd,
registered at the United Kingdom
Trade Marks Registry

DISTRIBUTORS

    Marston Book Services Ltd
    PO Box 269
    Abingdon, Oxon OX14 4YN
    (Orders: Tel: 01235 465500
            Fax: 01235 465555)

USA
    Blackwell Science, Inc.
    Commerce Place
    350 Main Street
    Malden, MA 02148-5018
    (Orders: Tel: 800 759 6102
            781 388 8250
        Fax: 781 388 8255)

Canada
    Login Brothers Book Company
    324 Saulteaux Crescent
    Winnipeg, Manitoba R3J 3T2
    (Orders: Tel: 204 837 2987

Australia
    Blackwell Science Pty Ltd
    54 University Street
    Carlton, Victoria 3053
    (Orders: Tel: 3 9347 0300
            Fax: 3 9347 5001)

A catalogue record for this title
is available from the British Library

ISBN 0-632-05039-X

Library of Congress
Cataloging-in-publication Data

The GP training handbook / edited by
    Michael Hall, Declan Dwyer, Tony
    Lewis. — 3rd ed.
        p.   cm.
    Includes bibliographical references.
    ISBN 0-632-05039-X
    1. Family medicine—Study and
teaching (Graduate)—Handbooks,
manuals, etc.
    2. Physicians (General practice)—
Training of—Handbooks, manuals, etc.
    3. Medical education—Handbooks,
manuals, etc.
    I. Hall, M.S.   II. Dwyer, Declan
III. Lewis, Tony.
    R840. G7   1999
    610′.71′1—dc21   98-40497
                                   CIP

For further information on
Blackwell Science, visit our website:
www.blackwell-science.com

Contents

Contributors iv

Foreword *Roger Neighbour* vii

Preface to the Third Edition xii

Preface to the First Edition xiii

1 Getting started *Jamie Bahrami and Helen Hall* 1

2 Hospital training *Christopher Hand* 14

3 Practice experience *John Salinsky* 29

4 The one-to-one tutorial *Tony Lewis* 53

5 Consultation skills *Peter Tate* 66

6 The vocational training scheme course *Russell Steele* 80

7 Preparing for summative assessment *Malcolm Campbell* 96

8 The MRCGP *Andrew Wilson* 119

9 Evidence-based practice in primary care
Trisha Greenhalgh 143

10 Audits, projects and research *John Sandars* 162

11 The practice as a small business within the NHS
Trisha Greenhalgh and Fraser Macfarlane 178

12 The trainer *Tim Swanwick* 195

13 Becoming a trainer *Mike Ruscoe* 213

14 Reading and writing *Domhnall MacAuley* 220

15 Practice systems *Terry Kemple* 235

16 Continuing your education *Paul Sackin* 252

Appendix 1: Directors and Deans of postgraduate GP
education (Regional Advisers) 274

Index 279

Contributors

Editors

Michael Hall FRCGP

Senior Lecturer (General Practice), Institute of General Practice, University of Exeter, School of Postgraduate Medicine and Health Sciences, Barrack Road, Exeter EX2 5DW

Declan Dwyer FDS FRCGP

Editor, *Education for General Practice*, Thurlestone, Devon TQ7 3NY

Tony Lewis FRCGP

General Practitioner, Regional Adviser (General Practice) for Devon and Cornwall, School of Postgraduate Medicine and Health Sciences, Barrack Road, Exeter EX2 5DW

Contributors

Jamie Bahrami MB ChB FRCOG FRCGP

Director of Postgraduate General Practice Education and Associate Dean for Yorkshire, Department for NHS Postgraduate Medical and Dental Education (Yorkshire), University of Leeds, Leeds LS2 9JT

Malcolm Campbell MB ChB DCH FRCGP

Assistant Director (Vocational Training), West of Scotland Postgraduate Medical Education Board, Honorary Clinical Senior Lecturer, Department of Postgraduate Medical Education, University of Glasgow, Glasgow G12 8QQ

Trisha Greenhalgh MA MD MRCP MRCGP

Senior Lecturer, Department of Primary Care and Population Sciences, University College of London Medical School / Royal Free Hospital of Medicine, Whittington Hospital, Highgate Hill, London N19 5NF

Helen Hall BA(Hons) MIPD

Head of Human Resources, UK Operations, BUPA, Staines, Middlesex TW18 4XF

Christopher Hand MAMSc MB BChir FRCGP MRCP

Associate Adviser (Postgraduate General Practice), Anglia and Oxford Region, Director and Honorary Senior Lecturer, General Practice Unit, School of Health Policy and Practice, University of East Anglia, Norwich NR4 7TJ

Terry Kemple

General Practitioner, Horfield Health Centre, Lockleaze Road, Horfield, Bristol BS7 9RR

Tony Lewis FRCGP

General Practitioner, Regional Adviser (General Practice) for Devon and Cornwall, School of Postgraduate Medicine and Health Sciences, Barrack Road, Exeter EX2 5DW

Domhnall MacAuley MD MRCGP MFPHM FISM

Professor of Primary Health Care, University of Ulster, Jordanstown, and Hillhead Family Practice, Belfast BT11 9FZ, Northern Ireland

Fraser Macfarlane BSc MBA MIHSM

Partner, Granville Sansom Personnel and Management Consultancy, Berkeley House, Barnet Road, London Colney, Herts AL2 1BG

Roger Neighbour MA MB BChir DObstRCOG FRCGP

Convenor, Panel of Examiners, Royal College of General Practitioners; Inaugural Fellow, Association of Course Organizers; Author, *The Inner Consultation* and *The Inner Apprentice*; Argowan, Bell Lane, Bedmond, Herts WD5 0QS

Mike Ruscoe FRCGP

General Practitioner, Associate Adviser (General Practice) for Devon and Cornwall, and MRCGP Examiner, Manor Surgery, Chapel Street, Redruth, Cornwall TR15 1AU

Paul Sackin FRCGP

General Practitioner and Course Organizer, Cambridge VTS, The Surgery, Alconbury, Huntingdon, Cambs PE17 5EQ

John Salinsky MA MRCP FRCGP

General Practitioner, Course Organizer, Whittington VTS Scheme, Chalk Hill Health Centre, Wembley, Middlesex HA9 9BQ

John Sandars FRCGP MRCP(UK)

General Practitioner and Trainer, Examiner MRCGP, Wilmslow Road Medical Centre, 166 Wilmslow Road, Handforth, Wilmslow, Cheshire SK9 3LF

Russell Steele FRCGP

General Practitioner, Associate Adviser (General Practice) for Devon and Cornwall, St Leonard's Medical Practice, 34 Denmark Road, Exeter EX4 4RS

Tim Swanwick MA(Cantab) MBBS DRCOG DCH MRCGP

Trainer in General Practice, Vine House Health Centre, 87–89 High Street, Abbots Langley, Herts WD5 0AJ

Peter Tate MBBS FRCGP

General Practitioner, Convenor MRCGP Video Examination, Culham, Abingdon on Thames, Oxfordshire OX14 4NA

Andrew Wilson BSc MB BS FRCGP DRCOG

General Practitioner, Associate Dean, Department of Postgraduate General Practice, North Thames (West), Imperial College School of Medicine, Du Cane Road, London W12 0NN

Foreword

Vocational training has to be counted amongst the most marvellous of institutions—those that do not show their age; and amongst the most admirable of traditions—those that are not ashamed of their history.

Tradition: now *there's* a notion to be ambivalent about. Becoming any kind of doctor involves reconciling oneself to the fact that, while the details may change with every general election and every issue of the *BMJ*, the profession of medicine and the ways of learning it are embedded in a cultural legacy going back unbroken for twenty-five centuries. If by 'tradition' we were to mean the intellectual equivalent of curare, a paralysing influence blocking adaptation and innovation, it would be a shackle rightly to be discarded. But to acknowledge the very best of our traditions can be to feel the comforting arm of history around our shoulders, and to hear the whispering voices of colleagues who, but for the accident of their decease, would still be on hand to say, '*If I could make a suggestion . . .*'

Take, for example, the idea of an educational contract, a statement of the terms and conditions on which a Registrar agrees to try and learn and a trainer agrees to try and help. Tim Swanwick in his chapter on the trainer (p. 199) underlines how empowering it is for the ground-rules of such an intense relationship to be made clear at its outset. He quotes work by Nick Foreman, who in turn canvassed his fellow Course Organizers as they formulated this principle in our contemporary language of aims, objectives, paradigms and learning styles. Here, it seems, a new and valuable tradition is being formed before our eyes. Nonetheless (and I see it as an endorsement, not a detraction), we might recall that the importance of setting an educational frame around clinical practice was first appreciated by Hippocrates. Some parts of his famous Oath (in Lloyd, 1978), such as foreswearing abortion, are now conveniently forgotten. Others we maintain we have risen above; we unconvincingly claim, for example, no longer to regard our stone-cutting urological surgical colleagues as *infra dig*. But Hippocrates, in his preamble before getting down to the clinical specifics, is quite clear. He requires the aspiring physician to swear '*by Apollo the physician, and Aesculapius, and Hygieia, and Panacea that I will keep this stipulation—to reckon him who taught me this Art equally dear to me as my parents, to share my substance with him, and relieve his necessities if required; to look upon his offspring in the same footing as my own brothers, and to teach them this art, if they shall wish to learn it, without fee or stipulation; and that by precept, lecture, and every other mode of instruction, I will impart a knowledge of the Art to my own sons, and those of my teachers, and to disciples bound by oath according to the law of medicine.*'

Make suitable sexist allowances, substitute Regional Director for Apollo, Aesculapius *et al.*, change '*share my substance*' to '*buy the odd beer*', and delete '*without fee*', and most of us would still sign up. The love of teaching, Hippocrates' sense that to hand on our hard-won skills is a privilege and a responsibility, still grabs us across the millennia.

C.P. Snow, in his 'two cultures' Rede lectures of 1959, recognized the sneering antagonism that had developed between science and art, our future prospects and the inheritance of the past. General practice sometimes aspires to be a *third* culture, one of 'all things to all men'. (Or so most patients expect and every government requires—and we willingly collude.) At all events, thoughtful commentators such as Iona Heath (1995) and James Willis (1995) evoke hankerings for a 'golden age' where the boundaries between thinking, knowing and supposing had not yet been marked out in barbed wire.

We could put an actual date to this mythic state of grace. It was over by 399 BC, when most of the writings of the Hippocratic school were complete and Socrates had been put to death for crimes against slipshod thinking.

Socrates and Hippocrates were the pioneers respectively of evidence-based philosophy and evidence-based medicine. In daily domestic and civil life theirs was a time of dialectic between speculation and observation, between rhetoric and logic. Rationality prevailed. Thereafter Western civilization committed itself to the view that the world could be studied more reliably with the

eyes open than with them closed. Not that the task was easy at
first: the early Hippocratic physicians had to work hard to per-
suade their contemporaries that, given the brevity of life itself, the
'craft so long to learn' was worth the learning. Diagnosis and
prognosis, cornerstones of practice then as now, were devised primarily as techniques to impress the patient and to disarm bereaved
and litigious next of kin. *Plus ça change?*

Whatever their motivation, Hippocrates and his followers
insisted that clinical practice required systematic and meticulous
observation. The treatise *Tradition in Medicine* (in Lloyd, 1978) is a
call for methodological rigour, recognizing the potential inexact-
ness of medical science and the weakness of theories based on
untestable hypotheses. The correspondences between Hippocratic tradition and our own professional values remain deep and
true. In them we can discern the origins of the modern medical
mind-set, the inculcation of which still remains the goal of contemporary vocational training.

But if Hippocrates has bequeathed to us the 'what', what of the
'how'?

The educational processes whereby Registrars are instructed
in, and inducted into, the profession of general practice also flow
from a vigorous traditional lineage, traceable back to the medieval
craft guilds. I have explored elsewhere (Neighbour, 1992) the
isomorphisms between the laborious progress of a 14th-century
would-be goldsmith from apprentice to journeyman to master-
craftsman and the fast-track equivalent of today's GP Registrar.
Both involve a complex 'relationship of tutelage' which, for all
its exhilaration and reward, is beset with objectives, curricula,
protocols, paradigms, rubrics and assessments. There has been in
some quarters a nostalgic reaction against this paraphernalia of
'education by formula' in favour of a return to 'learning by osmo-
sis' and 'seat of the pants' teaching. But this too has its dangers.

The work of general practice, like the visual arts, requires its
many dimensions and subtleties to be perceived all at once, unlike
literature or music which unfold sequentially in the linear flow of
time. The artist Paul Klee, lecturing in 1924, reminded his audience that the elements and techniques of visual art must be studied separately without losing sight of the fact that they are parts
of a whole. '*Otherwise*,' he asserted, '*our courage may fail us when we*

find ourselves faced with a new part leading in a completely different direction, into other dimensions, perhaps into a remoteness where the recollection of previously explored dimensions may easily fade' (in Herbert, 1964).

This is the courage required for training. It is the courage of the Arthurian Sir Gawain seeking the Holy Grail; of Tolkien's Bilbo Baggins; of Siegfried in Wagner's *Ring of the Nibelung* (and perhaps of those who listen to it!). For in vocational training, as in other tales of quest, it is not enough to reach the treasure; one must bring it back. It is not enough to benefit from the tradition, nor even to flourish under its governance; we are called upon to add to it. The art historian Roger Lipsey puts it this way (Lipsey, 1989): *'In any good teaching studio, today and always, mentors and their pupils are seized at moments by the archetypal pattern: differences in age, technical skill and sophistication of sensibility catalyse it. What is missing in our time is not richly endowed people to live the initiatic adventure but a clearer sense of tradition.'*

Hippocrates himself anticipated the travails awaiting his descendants. I have already alluded to the first of his *Aphorisms* (in Lloyd, 1978), beginning, *'Life is short, the craft so long to learn'*. It continues, *'Opportunity is elusive, experiment is dangerous, judgement is difficult.'* The authors of this book are all individuals who in their own clinical and educational lives have devoted themselves to the quest for mastery, found the courage, added to the tradition. Theirs are safe hands. They understand the component parts which they severally describe and the whole which they corporately reinforce. The reader who engages with them must take a chance, for the price of exposure to genuine authority is the risk of self-doubt. That risk is softened by the prospect of professional and intellectual renewal; and, as the composer Igor Stravinsky remarked, *'A renewal is fruitful only when it goes hand in hand with tradition.'*

Roger Neighbour

References

Heath, I. (1995) *The Mystery of General Practice*. Nuffield Provincial Hospitals Trust.

Herbert, R.L. (1964) *Modern Artists on Art*. Raven Press, Englewood Cliffs, NJ.

Lipsey, R. (1989) *An Art of Our Own: the Spiritual in Twentieth Century Art*. Shambhala, Boston, MA.

Lloyd, G.E.R. (1978) *Hippocratic Writings*. Penguin Classics.

Neighbour, R. (1992) *The Inner Apprentice*. Petroc Press, Newbury, UK.

Willis, J. (1995) *The Paradox of Progress*. Radcliffe Medical Press, Abingdon, UK.

Preface to the Third Edition

The new editorial team of *The GP Training Handbook* has been able to draw together leading general practice teachers to present a completely revised Third Edition. It covers all aspects of training, including the new arrangements for the membership examination of the RCGP. We hope the editorial style is easy to read and the book will serve as both a handbook for general practice trainers and registrars, as well as providing a useful reference book for those involved with general practice and masters degree courses.

We expect the handbook to be used as a reference text. For that reason, we make no apology for the occasional overlap between chapters which we believe makes it easier for readers who only refer to one particular aspect of training at a time.

Once again, the book appears at a time of great change in primary care. The advent of Primary Care Commissioning Groups gives much responsibility and a great opportunity to general practitioners, nurses and patients to help ensure that primary care in the NHS is strengthened and more able to provide the services which patients deserve. A sound and comprehensive training is therefore a pre-requisite and the new edition of this popular handbook will, we know, become a useful addition to the literature of general practice.

The editors wish to pay special thanks to Julie Orr for handling and collating the manuscripts.

Michael Hall
Declan Dwyer
Tony Lewis
February 1999

Preface to the First Edition

The idea of this book was conceived at a study weekend of doctors interested in the organization of general practice training in Devon and Cornwall and Oxford. All those involved in its production are active general practitioner (GP) teachers and face the day to day problems of running practices and teaching trainees. They are busy doctors and because of this they saw the need for a book offering practical help to colleagues in similar situations.

This handbook should therefore be the kind of book which you and your trainee can pick up and use at any time during the training period. It contains reference material on how to start preparing yourself to become a trainer and outlines changes which may need to be made in your practice amongst your partners or staff and your patients. It does not claim to be comprehensive, but is aimed at stimulating trainers to search for ways of improving both their medical practice and their standard of teaching. A simple practical approach has been adopted. We have tried to avoid lengthy theoretical discussion.

We also believe that the literature of general practice has grown so rapidly that it would be unfair of us to attempt to impose our beliefs and we suggest throughout the text further reading for those who wish.

We have paid particular attention to the creation of a practical assessment scheme. There are lots of simple checklists from which trainers and trainees may select those most suitable to their needs.

Most of us are members of the Royal College of General Practitioners (RCGP), by examination. Readers will not be surprised, therefore, to see that we believe that the MRCGP examination has an important place at the end of a time of preparation for general practice. A trainer, whether or not a member of the RCGP, has a responsibility to inform his trainee about the 'nuts and bolts' of the examination and to offer help in preparing for it. Since experiencing an examination is an excellent way of learning about it, we suggest that all trainers should sit the MRCGP examination.

The section about teaching in the practice describes the commonly used techniques and explores the potential of the practice as an educational arena. Developing a skill in the consultation comes not just with experience but with an understanding of what happens between doctor and patient when they consult together. The project is presented as an opportunity for the trainee to consider in depth a particular aspect of general practice and to learn by handling information for himself. Case discussion is the very centre of general practice training and we describe various teaching methods using the mass of material presented in any record of a consultation.

Trainees are demanding more formal teaching within their training practices. In Chapter 16 we offer a tutorial guide, showing what to teach and some questions to ask. We cannot claim that all of general practice is covered by our topics but we believe that if every trainer could discuss at least half the topics listed during the course of a traineeship there would be few complaints from trainees of inadequate teaching.

Because advances and changes in medical practice follow with such rapidity we believe that no set of textbooks can keep any one doctor fully up to date. Doctors must develop their own information base and to this end we recommend that each doctor keep a file of information parallel with each of the headings listed in the tutorial guide. Clearly, such a file will reflect the doctors own particular interest but it can be updated by a trainee working up a topic.

Trainees have a splendid opportunity during their training year to build up their own reference base, both of data acquired at the vocational training course, in the practices and elsewhere. The example set by the trainer is one of the most potent influences on the future educational and professional behaviour of the doctor in training. The trainer's responsibility is considerable. The future pattern of general practice will depend in the main on the attitudes instilled in a trainee during his training year.

Good teachers are usually enthusiasts for their subject. The emphasis in any one trainer–trainee pairing will be different from the next but having 'the right tools to do the job' will ensure that the quality of the learning is the best possible. To this end, enthu-siasm needs to be matched with good medical records, a good library and an understanding practice staff. From such a basis great deeds can be done. We hope you will enjoy our book as much as you enjoy medicine and teaching medicine.

MSH

1982

1 Getting started

Let us assume you have considered all your options and decided on a career in general practice. Now, all you want to know is how to get started. This chapter explains the vocational training system and the factors that you will have to take into account in planning your training.

Vocational training regulations

In accordance with the Regulations (NHS, 1979, 1998), the training programme should consist of a minimum 24 months in educationally approved and specially selected posts, normally at senior house officer (SHO) level, and 12 months in general practice. The posts at preregistration house officer level are not acceptable for the purpose.

Prescribed experience

Ideally, you should plan your training in such a way that it would follow the standard format called 'prescribed experience'. The details of prescribed experience are summarized in Box 1.1.

Equivalent experience

If your training programme does not fully comply with the requirements of prescribed experience, or one of the posts that you completed was more than 7 years ago, then you can apply to the Joint Committee on Postgraduate Training for General Practice (JCPTGP) for your experience to be considered under the terms of 'equivalent experience' (Box 1.2).

Please remember, in the first instance, you should always discuss your training requirement with the director of postgraduate general practice education for the region in which you want to

---

Box 1.1 Prescribed experience

- Training is undertaken in the UK and should total not less than 36 months whole-time employment or the equivalent part time
- Is completed within the 7-year period immediately preceding application for a certificate
- Includes, at least, 12 months full-time employment or its equivalent part time as a GP registrar within the NHS
- Includes training in hospital or community medicine posts which have been specifically approved for general practice training, including not less than 6 months whole-time employment, or the equivalent part time in each of two of the following listed specialties: general medicine, geriatric medicine, paediatrics, psychiatry, accident and emergency or general surgery, obstetrics or gynaecology, or obstetrics and gynaecology

---

Box 1.2 Equivalent experience

- Posts must have appropriate educational content with appropriate supervision
- Overseas posts must have been inspected and approved locally with an appropriate recognized training authority
- Posts in the EU must have had approval status for general practice training in that country
- The mix of posts must be relevant to general practice
- Experience for a certificate of equivalent experience should normally be acquired within the 10-year period immediately preceding the date of application
- There must be continuity of clinical contact or activity throughout the 10-year period

---

train. The names and addresses of directors and the address of the JCPTGP appear in Appendix 1.

Full time or part time

Your general practice training can be completed either full time or part time, or even as a mixture of the two. The choice is largely yours and depends on your social/domestic situation and preferences. The part-time training (now called flexible training) needs

---

Box 1.3 Flexible training

- The total duration of training is not shortened
- The weekly duration of part-time training is not less than 60% of full-time training
- There shall be some full-time training periods (in both hospital and general practice). This can be a minimum of only two periods of full-time employment of not less than 1 week in each component of training
- The quality of training experienced must be equivalent to that in full-time training

Note: As a consequence of this change, your general practice component of training will therefore be 20 months at 60% instead of the previous 24 months at 50%. Similarly, the hospital component of training will be 40 months instead of the previous 48 months at 50%.

---

to be carefully planned and discussed with the deanery in which you plan your training. Also, this will have to comply with the European Union (EU) Directive 93/16/EEC, which is summarized in Box 1.3.

Two ways of training

There are two ways of training. You can either choose to join a vocational training scheme or you can construct your own training programme. Which is better? Joining a scheme offers many advantages that are not readily available in self-constructed programmes. These are summarized in Box 1.4.

Box 1.4 Some of the advantages of a scheme

- A scheme offers you a package of appropriate posts in various specialties and general practice
- A scheme will give you the benefit of professional support by course organizers and their colleagues
- You will join a peer group of GP registrars
- A scheme offers you specific educational programmes, e.g. half-day release
- Above all, a scheme provides you with stability

Some other features of a scheme

Generally, the scheme is district-based and in close proximity to a trust hospital. The core structure of the scheme consists of a range of appropriately selected specialty or community posts, usually at SHO level. In addition, the scheme has many training practices that have been specially selected and approved for training. Although most of the schemes are similar in structure, there are some individual variations, which give each scheme its own identity and character.

These variations may include:

Range and choice of posts

Some schemes offer you a very fixed set of rotations at the point of entry. It is usually difficult to change your rotation or swap one particular post for another at a later date. Other schemes tend to be more flexible and take note of your educational needs and can change your rotation as appropriate. Some of the more forward-looking schemes have now moved away from the rigid structure of the past and offer a modular approach to training. This means that you will have a broader experience of specialties in a shorter period of time, usually from a base in general practice. However, even in these schemes, the rotations on offer must fully satisfy the requirements of vocational training regulations.

Attitude

There are differences in attitude in each scheme towards GP registrars and their training. Some tend to be more registrar-centred and allow time and space for your professional development. The educational programmes of these schemes are heavily influenced by your needs. As a result, the half-day-release course generally uses the problem-solving model, in which peer group learning is encouraged and pastoral care is an essential element. The other schemes, in contrast, may have a more formal approach to learning, such as the use of a well-defined core curriculum over a 3-year period. This has the disadvantage that, if you enter the scheme at a 'wrong' time, i.e. outside the normal cycle, you could miss part of the curriculum!

Admittedly, in an ideal scheme, there should be a healthy mixture of the two, avoiding extremes and relying more on an adult learning model (Brookfield, 1986). This will allow you to take responsibility for your own learning. This means that you should be aware of your own attitude to learning, which may have been coloured adversely by your previous experiences. Do not worry if this is the case, but be prepared to be flexible and open to new influences and ideas.

Locality

Another important factor which, to a certain extent, affects the educational profile of the scheme is its locality. In an inner-city-based vocational training scheme, the learning priorities may be influenced more by the problems of an inner-city conurbation than by those of a rural environment. For example, problems of drug misuse, socioeconomic issues and deprivation statistics could dominate the learning agenda. If you are totally committed to a general practice career in a different environment to that of the scheme, then there could be a mismatch of expectations between you and the scheme. However, you should bear in mind that, as a GP, you can never totally escape a particular problem in which you have no interest. Believe it or not, even in a seemingly idyllic rural practice, you may still be faced with socioeconomic problems!

In choosing a training scheme, consider the factors described below.

You

Your attitude to medicine and general practice as a career

Do you see medicine/general practice as a vocation, or a job which has to be done competently and well without sacrificing personal and private life?

Your preferred style of learning

We all have different and preferred learning styles. It is important to know that and to choose the scheme or training programme which, in general, offers you the most appropriate response.

Do you intend to pursue higher professional education, for example, academic/research?
If you do, then clearly you have to choose a scheme and locality where such opportunities exist.

Where do you wish to settle after your training?
When you train in a particular locality, you will establish contacts and get to know the system. Therefore, it will be easier for you to find a suitable practice to join. So choose a scheme in a locality which is likely to be your resting place!

Your previous educational and cultural experiences
These may have some effect on your expectation of learning. You should be prepared to explore these and discuss them with colleagues, course organizers or other key people in the training network.

The scheme

The following features of the scheme should be considered:
- The attitude of key players in the scheme, which should always be positive and enthusiastic.
- The track record of the scheme.
- The structure and options that it offers should match your expectations.
- The learning model of the scheme must be in tune with your learning style.
- The scheme should ideally exhibit flexibility rather than rigidity.
- The geography of the scheme, such as ease of access to centres of excellence in training, must be considered.
- Members of the scheme should be approachable, helpful, tolerant and compassionate.
- The scheme should be offering you regular opportunities for appraisal, counselling and mentoring.

Action

You should start finding out all there is to know about the scheme by seeking information from the course organizer and/or his/ her administrative staff. Most will have printed information and some can supply a video describing the scheme. You should attempt to:

- Meet the past and present registrars to find out what they thought was good and what, in their opinion, was unsatisfactory about the scheme.
- Arrange an appointment to see the course organizer to discuss your expectations and also judge his or her attitude to general practice training and you.
- Visit one or two training practices and talk to some of the trainers and staff in both hospital and general practice posts.

After each encounter, make a note about what you have heard and, more significantly, what you have not heard!

Self-constructed programme of training

A second way of training is to construct your own programme. Some 50% of GP registrars plan their own programme. You may wonder, in view of the obvious advantages of a scheme, why they choose to do this. The reasons are varied. Some registrars may not be sure about their career intentions until later on, by which time they could have completed a few hospital posts. Others may experience domestic pressures which would make it impossible for them to commit themselves for any particular length of time to a particular location.

Beware...!! There is nothing inherently wrong with a self-constructed programme of training, as long as you remember the following points:

- Discuss your plan with somebody who knows the system, for example the director of postgraduate general practice education.
- Find out if your previous experience is acceptable for general practice training (contact the director or the Joint Committee).
- Select only those posts which are approved for general practice training. The director's office can verify the status of each post.

- Even though you are not on a scheme, immediately contact the local course organizer and get involved in general practice training courses and activities.

How do you select the general practice post?

Regardless of whether you are on a scheme or self-constructed programme of training, you will require a minimum of 12 months in a general practice post or posts as a registrar. All training practices are part and parcel of the scheme and, in accordance with the Joint Committee policy, all appointments to the practice must be made through the scheme. Therefore, although you may be aware of a particular vacancy in a training practice, or a training practice that you prefer, you should always approach the course organizer in the first instance.

What you should know about training practices

The points you should be aware of are summarized in Box 1.5.

What you can claim as a GP registrar

These details are spelt out in the Statement of Fees and Allowances (the 'Red Book'), and have been summarized in Box 1.6.

Your decision

Once you have all the information, take some time to complete your checklist, and reflect on what you have learned and what you still need to learn. If there is nothing further that you need to know, then **make a final decision and please stick to it**.

A reassuring fact

If all this sounds too daunting, there is at least one reassuring fact that you should bear in mind. That is, all the schemes and practices provide a satisfactory standard of training, otherwise they would not have been approved by the JCPTGP.

Box 1.5 Some essential elements of a training practice

- Only 10% of practitioners in the UK are trainers
- Trainers and their practices are selected in accordance with a very strict set of criteria, decided by the JCPTGP
- Training practices are monitored regularly, at least every 3 years, by an inspection visit on behalf of the deanery (the new title for region!)
- Trainers are trained teachers
- You are supernumerary in the practice
- You will not be exploited for service commitment at the expense of your education
- You will have continuing appraisal/counselling in the practice
- You will have a written contract of employment with the practice. This covers hours of work, study leave, maternity and sick leave and holiday entitlement. It should also explain the duties and responsibilities of the trainer and the registrar

Box 1.6 What you can claim as a GP registrar

- Car allowance, currently £3730 a year, but taxable
- Removal and related accommodation expenses
- Sickness payments for absence of less than 3 months
- Entitlement to paid maternity leave
- Travelling and subsistence allowances for sitting examinations for postgraduate qualifications

But also remember, applying blindly to a scheme or a post, without proper consideration of all the above factors, can lead to a very unhappy period of training. The time for training is short, and you do not want to waste it by being dissatisfied and frustrated. Therefore, time spent in finding out about the posts and the people involved is definitely worthwhile.

Make sure you suit the post and the post suits you.

A few tips about your application

Having gone to all the trouble of finding the ideal scheme or practice, it would be a great pity if you did not get the job that you wanted for lack of attention to your application. If you have time, please peruse through one or two books (Jackson, 1991; Yate, 1992) and consult with experienced colleagues.

The final section of this chapter is designed to help you construct a CV which promotes you in the best possible way.

Preparing a CV

Once you have decided to pursue your career in general practice, you will begin researching suitable schemes and planning your application approach.

In any job search, preparation will be the key aid in sending out a good self-marketing personal document demonstrating your skills, experience and strengths.

There are a number of factors that influence those who screen CVs on a regular basis in positive selection. In that respect it will be worth following some general pointers.

However, you must remember that your CV is selling you, it should reflect your personality. While this section gives a number of guidelines and helpful hints, you must select the format that suits you and best displays your skills and achievements.

What is the CV?

Your CV should be a personal document promoting you. Its purpose is not to secure you a job but rather to enable you to get an interview. It should give an account of you, with clear examples of your knowledge, experience and skills.

Preparation

In preparing your CV you need to plan what you want from your training scheme. Later chapters describe a number of variations in different schemes. Therefore, once you have decided which aspects are important to you, your CV will need to be tailored accordingly.

The preparation which you put in at this stage will be invaluable at any interviews you are invited to attend. You should not commence drafting your CV until you have:
- Researched, understood and decided what you want from a training scheme (and general practice career thereafter).

- Understood and can justify with practical examples your key skills and strengths.

In a CV you do not refer to your weaknesses, but you must have some insight into what they are and how you are addressing them, as this is a legitimate area for questioning in an interview.

Style and layout

For those who read through a large number of CVs the style and layout are crucial. Lengthy, wordy documents do not make life easy for those selecting, and your CV may end up in the 'Reject' pile for the wrong reasons. The following suggestions are agreed 'best practice' guidelines:

- Keep your CV to one page, maximum two.
- Ensure it is not cramped, but easy to read.
- List all personal details first.
- Use active, descriptive verbs.
- Remove all irrelevant information and surplus words as they reduce impact.
- Leave generous margins to break up the text.
- Include a 'profile statement' in bold.

Content

When assembling personal information and facts you will almost certainly end up with more than you need to use. However, this will not be wasted information and it is likely that it will be used at the interview stage.

A profile statement has become a popular key addition to CVs; it should be a short, snappy paragraph which summarizes your key skills and personal qualities (see Box 1.7). It should begin with

---

Box 1.7 Example of a profile statement

An enthusiastic vocationally trained family physician with additional experience in care of the elderly and public health medicine. Special interest in practice organization and personal and staff career development

your current title (i.e. GP registrar) and should be relevant to the post for which you are applying. In some instances this may be the only part of the CV which is read properly.

Once you have gathered all of your information, structure it around the headings set out in Box 1.8, omitting any surplus, irrelevant facts. This structure will then form the content of your CV.

Box 1.8 Summary of CV requirements

- Personal details
- Profile statement
- Qualifications (with dates)
- Current appointments, experience and achievements
- Previous appointments, experience and achievements
- Relevant areas of interest (keep to a minimum)
- Any research or publications

Helpful hints

The following are additional hints which, as a result of your CV, should help to gain you an interview:
- Do not attach photographs (unless specifically requested).
- Do not put the CV in a binder or wallet, use a paperclip or staple or treasury tag.
- Use quality A4 paper, do not send photocopies.
- Too much detail and information on hobbies distracts from the main purpose.
- Omit any personal information that is not relevant to the job.
- Ensure it is error-free, check thoroughly for spelling and grammatical mistakes.

The covering letter

You should always include a covering letter with your CV. While it is useful to have a standard draft letter, remember to customize it to suit your application. Today these letters are usually typed, but some prospective employers request handwritten letters.

The format and content of the letter could be as follows:
1 Restate what you believe they are looking for. Confirm you have understood the position by demonstrating your research and understanding of the practice setting.
2 Include two or three key skills or achievements which make you suitable.
3 State the benefits you could bring—as a result of your knowledge, skills or experience.
4 Confirm your serious interest in the post, express a wish to find out more information. Confirm your availability for interview.

Remember

- No negative statements.
- No reasons for leaving previous jobs.
- Do not include salary requirements.
- Check spelling and grammar.

References

Brookfield, S.D. (1986) *Understanding and Facilitating Adult Learning.* Open University Press, Milton Keynes.

Jackson, T. (1991) *The Perfect CV.* Piatkus, London.

NHS (1979, 1998) *NHS Vocational Training Regulations.* HMSO, London.

Yate, M.J. (1992) *Great Answers to Tough Interview Questions.* Kogan Page, New York.

2 Hospital training

Introduction

How does training in hospital relate to training for general practice? It does seem very strange that three of the four years of GP training should be spent in a hospital environment. It is all the more surprising now that much of the training of medical students occurs in the community and more care is being shifted from secondary to primary care. Unfortunately, there is a long way to go before the educational needs of future GPs are seen to be of equal importance to the training needs of hospital specialists and the service needs of secondary care. The Royal College of General Practitioners (RCGP), despite representing half of the medical profession, is only one college among several longer-established colleges involved in the training of doctors. Furthermore, GP training is controlled by legislation and, although this has recently changed, the funding arrangements for training have not. This situation is hindering progress.

First this chapter briefly describes how the present situation has developed. Then the current training position and how to get the best out of training in hospital is described in more detail. Finally, suggestions are made about how we might use hospitals more selectively for GP training in the future.

History

The first of the College Reports from General Practice, published in 1965, proposed a broadly based programme containing several hospital posts with GP training (Pereira Gray, 1992). The following year, the College published its evidence to the Royal Commission on Medical Education and recommended a minimum period of 4 years training after registration—2 years in hospital and 2 years in supervised general practice. This was accepted, and when the Todd Report was published in 1968 it introduced the concept of general professional training that was to be undertaken over a 5-year period, which included the preregistration year. The Vocational Training Regulations that were passed by Act of Parliament in 1976 stipulated only a 3-year programme, of which 18 months could be taken in general practice. In reality, because of difficulties in funding the extra 6 months in general practice and the need to provide a service in hospitals, 2 years' training in hospital became the norm.

The early vocational training schemes in Scotland, Wessex and East Anglia were based at district general hospitals and included 6-month rotations. These rotations comprised various combinations of paediatrics, obstetrics and gynaecology, medicine, accident and emergency, psychiatry and other minor specialties. Half-day release or, in some fortunate districts, whole-day release continued throughout the two hospital years, so that some continuity in training for general practice was provided.

Current situation

The basic structure of GP training has changed remarkably little in the past 20 years, and most training schemes are the same as the early model described above. Schemes, however, do vary in the way the general practice year is organized. Some schemes take the whole year in practice after the 2 years in hospital posts has been completed Other schemes split the year into: 1 month and 11 months; 3 months and 9 months; or equally into 6 months. There are definite advantages in taking some of the general practice component before starting on the 2 years in hospital. The most obvious advantage is that the experience in general practice can be used to guide the education obtained in hospital. GP registrars who undertake an introductory period in general practice are more likely to consider that they receive relevant teaching from hospital staff (Crawley & Levin, 1990).

The arrival of summative assessment in September 1997 may well herald changes in the introductory period. The year in general practice is now so full that obtaining the four components of summative assessment, let alone taking the MRCGP examination, makes it more likely that the year in practice will be taken at the end of training. Short introductory periods may remain, but the problem with this arrangement is that the start date of the senior house officer (SHO) post is out of phase with other posts in the hospital.

The preregistration year

One possible way around this problem is to obtain some general practice experience in the preregistration year, rather than doing the traditional 6 months medicine and 6 months surgery. Schemes offering 4 months in general practice have been available for over 10 years, but they are by no means common. Unfortunately, they **were** limited by the requirements of Section 12 of the Medical Act 1983, restricting the approval of general practices for general clinical training to those located in publicly owned health centres (General Medical Council, Education Subcommittee, 1997). **These regulations, however, were changed in 1997 and have been applied from August 1998**.

Minor surgery skills can also be learnt in the preregistration year and there is evidence that the educational potential of surgical house officer posts is not exploited (Pringle *et al.*, 1991).

Training schemes and the day-release programme

The big advantage of joining a formal training scheme is that it provides job security for 3 years and that the day-release programme usually runs throughout the hospital component as well. Historically, attendance at the release courses has been a problem in many hospitals, with GP registrars in some specialties having particular difficulty (Crawley & Levin, 1990). Constructing one's own scheme does provide more job flexibility. Most GP registrars, however, want the same training experience, with medicine, obstetrics, paediatrics and dermatology being considered the most relevant specialties by those who have had experience of them (Kelly & Murray, 1991). Registrars constructing their own scheme are usually unable to attend the day-release programme, which is a major disadvantage, as someone has to cover the wards for colleagues who are on the scheme.

Some schemes have tackled the problem of attendance at the

day-release course by organizing their courses in blocks of a week rather than on single days or half-days. The advantage of this approach is that hospital management can organize locum cover well in advance, and this may enable registrars constructing their own scheme to attend the course. The main disadvantage is that the protected weekly contact with GP peers and course organizers is lost.

The Joint Committee on Postgraduate Training for General Practice regulations

The new regulations relating to the hospital component of GP training came into force on 30 January 1998. They are complex and determined by the NHS (Vocational Training for General Medical Practice) Regulations 1997. The reader would be well advised to consult the latest edition of *A Guide to Certification*, published by the Joint Committee on Postgraduate Training for General Practice (JCPTGP), which explains the regulations in detail.

In summary, the regulations specify two types of experience: prescribed and equivalent. Prescribed experience is training that follows the standard format. This usually consists of 2 years (whole time or the equivalent part time) in what are known as short-list posts. The posts are in those specialties that contain the knowledge and experience most GPs will need during their careers as generalists. The specialties are:
- general medicine
- geriatric medicine
- paediatrics (this means medical paediatrics)
- psychiatry
- one of accident and emergency medicine; or general surgery; or accident and emergency medicine and general surgery; or accident and emergency medicine and orthopaedic surgery
- one of obstetrics; or gynaecology; or obstetrics and gynaecology.

The majority of schemes are made up of these posts, usually four 6-month posts. It is also possible to obtain prescribed experience by doing a maximum of 6 months in other specialties relevant to general practice; some training schemes include combinations of minor specialties, such as 3 months' ophthalmology and 3 months' ear, nose and throat.

GP registrars who organize their own schemes must spend at least 1 year in short-list posts and they will be expected to have done at least two of these posts. The maximum period in any one specialty that can be counted towards the hospital component of their training programme is now 12 months. If they choose they can make up the other year with what are commonly know as middle-year posts. Middle-year posts include experience in those minor specialties that GPs might find useful. Spending a whole 2 years in hospital doing these jobs might be considered to provide an unbalanced training, which is why only 1 year is permitted. Although the regulations allow for this middle year to be spent in general practice, funding is not normally available. Depending on what combination of posts is taken, certificates of either prescribed or equivalent experience will be granted.

The new regulations give the JCPTGP the responsibility of approving all hospital posts for GP training. The first step in the process is approval by the Specialist Training Authority of the Medical Royal Colleges (STA). The second step is for the deanery general practice education committee to identify posts suitable for GP training. Posts that are not educationally approved as prescribed experience, but which the education committee feels are suitable for GP training, are presented to the JCPTGP for equivalent experience. The JCPTGP grants the final approval, but it also has the authority to withdraw it.

There are two traps into which unwary GP registrars constructing there own courses can fall. The first, which is happening more often, is when a post changes as a result of reorganization within a trust. If a post changes in any way, then it must be reconsidered by the education committee and then submitted to the JCPTGP. Unfortunately, this does not always happen. The second trap is when the registrar takes a post that is a combination of minor specialties. These posts do not have either STA approval (normally a minimum of 6 months for specialist training) or JCPTGP approval for prescribed experience.

If a post is not approved for equivalent or prescribed experience, then the registrar has to apply personally to the JCPTGP for retrospective approval under equivalent experience. While it is probable that they will get equivalent experience, it is best for them to get advice before they start the post. This advice applies equally to those who have worked in hospital posts outside the UK.

The education committee does not select posts that are too specialized and unsuitable for GP training. An example would be renal medicine, where most of the work is with patients on dialysis. Registrars constructing their own scheme can still apply for retrospective experience for these posts and a proportion, say 3 months, might be allowed towards the 2-year hospital training component. This situation usually occurs with doctors who have changed career from hospital medicine to general practice. These doctors are well advised to consult their GP director and the JCPTGP about their general practice training needs in advance.

At the end of each post, the GP registrar has to obtain a consultant's signature, the GP director's endorsement and the hospital stamp on a VTR2 form. This is a statement of competence as well as of attendance.

Monitoring visits

The responsibility for monitoring education and training was originally that of the royal colleges. The system of hospital visiting with specialty colleges joining forces with the RCGP is well established, but it does have problems (Hand, 1994). Monitoring educational standards is also the responsibility of the postgraduate deans, whose budgets contribute 100% of preregistration house officers' and 50% of the SHOs' salaries. The JCPTGP, which accredits GP training provided by regions, also inspects hospital posts. This cumbersome system leads to duplication of effort, and some regions are beginning to combine royal college and postgraduate dean visits. The visits are, however, an opportunity for junior doctors to discuss their training in confidence with people who are not involved with the progress of their careers. Questionnaires are usually sent out before the visits and can be especially useful in highlighting difficult issues. Several questionnaires are in current use, and it is important that they are both valid and reliable (Hand & Adams, 1998).

Box 2.1 Hard and soft criteria used by the RCGP for judging standards of hospital training

Hard (essential) criteria
• Contract of employment
• Clinical duties
• Duty rotas
• Induction course
• Domestic arrangements
• Educational supervisor
• Formative assessment
• Study leave
• Clinical back up
• Clinical experience
• Clinical discussions
• Library and postgraduate medical centre facilities
• Inappropriate routine tasks

Soft (optional) criteria
• Contractual educational experience
• Trained educational supervisor
• Childcare facilities
• System for pastoral needs
• Recreational facilities
• Valuing and supporting culture
• Structured system of assessment for VTR2

The criteria that the RCGP use for judging standards of hospital training are similar to those laid down by the General Medical Council (GMC) for preregistration house officers (General Medical Council, Education Subcommittee, 1997) and by the Academy of Royal Colleges for the training of senior house officers (Academy of Royal Colleges, 1997). The criteria are summarized in Box 2.1.

The new deal

The new deal for junior doctors (NHS Management Executive, 1991) means that SHOs should be on call for no more than 72 hours a week. Other European countries manage to train their doctors in a much less onerous fashion. In Denmark, Norway and Sweden, junior doctors work 37–45 hours a week and in the Netherlands they are limited to 48 hours. At least a quarter of British junior doctor posts failed to meet the deadline for the new deal in December 1996, with juniors still working more than 56 hours a week. Shorter working hours means an increased intensity of work and this can be extremely stressful. Although this is not a new phenomenon (Firth-Cozens, 1987), it is important that those who experience undue stress know where they can go for help, and others are aware that colleagues may be in trouble. Being registered with a GP is essential.

In one recent survey of 120 trusts, no one met the new deal criteria on accommodation and catering. Individual trusts, however, have made great strides in improving the lot of their junior doctors (Moore *et al.*, 1994), and this shows what can be achieved when doctors and managers work together. A good summary of the new deal can be found in the *Guide to House Jobs in Yorkshire*, which is published annually by the West Yorkshire Junior Doctors' Committee of the British Medical Association (Smith & Cummings, 1997). The production of such an excellent guide is an example that other regions would do well to follow.

Calman training

The implications of Calman training for specialists are only just beginning to be realized. There will be more training and less service work for junior doctors in a system that is to be more consultant-based than consultant-led. This change could well put pressure on GP registrars, in terms of both service commitment and attendance at release courses. Some integration of general professional training for specialists and GPs seems desirable, with core subjects, such as communication skills, clinical decision making, critical appraisal of evidence, health economics and medical ethics, being the common ground.

Many of the specialist royal colleges are organizing their SHO posts into 2-year rotations, with links being made between hospital trusts. This will reduce the choice of posts for registrars constructing their own scheme, as well as having a profound effect on training schemes.

Satisfaction with training

Several surveys have demonstrated that GPs are dissatisfied with many aspects of the training that they receive in hospitals (Reeve & Bowman, 1989; Little, 1994; Kelly & Murray, 1997). What is so disappointing is that this situation has not really changed for several years. The main criticisms are:
- an absence of educational objectives
- insufficient formal teaching
- little or no informal teaching
- teaching not orientated towards general practice
- inadequate feedback
- problems with study leave
- difficulty in attending GP day release
- lack of protected time for individual study.

There is some evidence that things may be improving for junior doctors (Paice *et al.*, 1997b), but whether this applies to those training for general practice is not known. Given these circumstances, what can be done?

Improving the educational experience

How to help the SHO get the best out of the post

Baker (1993) has suggested ways in which the educational content of SHO posts could be enhanced. These include:
- a named educational supervisor
- personal educational objectives
- logbooks
- formal assessment
- feedback on performance
- feedback to departments.

A named educational supervisor or mentor would enable the SHO to develop a closer relationship with one consultant. This has been shown to work well in general practice where GP registrars have an individual trainer. This arrangement should provide for better continuity of education, given the new working patterns in hospitals. Training for the role of supervisor should be provided, and ideally the work should be part of the consultant contract and separately remunerated.

With personal educational objectives, doctors are in a much better position to identify what they can learn from their day-to-day work (Grant & Marsden, 1989). Also having these objectives incorporated into a logbook can enhance the educational process (Paice *et al.*, 1997a). The RCGP has published educational objectives for hospital posts in conjunction with specialist colleges and associations, and these have been revised recently (see Further reading, p.28).

Seeing that objectives have been successfully met is an integral part of both summative assessment and formative appraisal. These processes are still not as widespread as they should be, mainly because consultants have not received the training required (Bunch *et al.*, 1997). The combined role of judge and mentor is not easy, and ideally the two roles should be separate. Given the number of consultants for whom most SHOs work, this should be possible. Furthermore, now that summative assessment for GP registrars is compulsory, some of the trainer's report could be completed during hospital training and the current VTR2 might become unnecessary. The educational supervisor's role would then be more one of co-ordination and guidance of education rather than assessment of competence.

Feedback on performance is as important for the learner as it is for the teacher. Formal appraisal halfway through the post and at the end should be the minimum in a 6-month post. There should be a mechanism whereby SHOs can give constructive feedback to the department on the quality of their training. The various hospital visiting systems provide one mechanism, but this is rather impersonal. The whole philosophy of giving honest feedback should be developed early in one's career and should be seen as the norm rather than the exception.

How to get the best out of your post

Educational experts emphasize that much of adult learning is both self-directed and problem-based. There are numerous learning opportunities in hospital, but a considerable amount of personal motivation and organization is needed in a busy post. Some excellent guidance on how to learn 'on the job' is now available for learners and teachers (see Further reading, p.28). Taking control of your learning is possible, and now you have permission!

How to co-ordinate hospital training with general practice training

In addition to running the day-release programme, GP course organizers have an important role in co-ordinating the hospital component of the scheme. Regular communication with consultants is essential, although the day-to-day practicalities of this are often difficult. Joint meetings between GP and hospital trainers occur in some regions and are a useful forum in which to discuss educational objectives and training problems.

In some districts, course organizers are involved in the formative appraisal process of GP registrars. Even if each course organizer is only responsible for six SHOs, this will still mean 24 meetings a year. Sharing the responsibility with GP trainers can lighten the load and provide some continuity with the training practice. With the present training regulations, the time involved is not funded unless the trainer has another GP registrar in post.

The future of hospital training for general practice

The pressures on general practice

Recruitment to general practice has been falling despite the pressure for a primary-care-led NHS. Unless the medicopolitical climate changes radically, this trend is likely to continue. With more doctors training to be specialists, the hospital service will be less dependent upon GPs to fill SHO posts.

Patient demand in general practice has increased and this need has been met partially by sharing work with other members of the primary health care team. More registrars in general practice might alleviate some of this pressure, especially if a second year in practice were allowed.

The changing roles of GPs

The 1990 Contract and the NHS reforms have produced challenges for GPs. The introduction of fundholding and, more recently, locality purchasing has required new skills. The shift of work from secondary to primary care has meant more responsibility for the management of chronic illness, both physical and mental. Midwives, on the other hand, now take on more obstetric care. These major changes mean that the balance of training between general practice and hospital medicine almost certainly needs to be revised.

The development of training for general practice

Short hospital rotations or special attachments?
The Royal College of General Practitioners (1994) has recommended 18 months training in hospital and 18 months in general practice. Ideally, short rotations of 3 or 4 months would enable a wider experience of specialties to be obtained. While this suggestion might not meet with consultant approval, the experience in other countries, such as the USA (R.M. Berrington, personal communication, 1997), shows that it can work well.

A more radical solution would be for all the training, except perhaps for the preregistration period, to be in general practice. GP educators would then purchase any hospital training that was required.

Multiprofessional learning and the role of universities
The newly established regional consortia, which have GP representation, are responsible for commissioning non-medical education and training. They also have a responsibility to advise about medical education. Co-ordination of medical and non-medical training and workforce planning is almost inevitable.

Learning with other health professionals is a logical extension of working in teams. Professional boundaries can be broken down and interprofessional relationships enhanced by sharing experiences in a neutral academic setting. Masters courses are springing up in universities all over the country and offer excellent opportunities for multiprofessional learning and research. In some places, hospital doctors are using these courses as part of their higher specialist (Calman) training.

With more of the education of health professionals taking place in partnership with universities, there is now an ideal opportunity to forge more effective links between education, research and development and audit. This would enable a culture of questioning clinical practice, searching for the evidence and putting it into practice. If this happened, then GPs could spend more time learning with their hospital colleagues rather than from them.

Conclusion

Training for general practice is about to enter a new phase of development, with more GP training taking place in the community and less emphasis being placed on training in hospital. Changes in the demands of general practice, as well as in the training of specialists, make this imperative. While this has major implications for running the hospital service, the problems are not insurmountable.

With the NHS moving from an era of competition to one of co-operation, it is hoped that the royal colleges will plan the education and training of their doctors together. In future, perhaps some of the training for hospital doctors will take place in general practice.

Acknowledgements

I would like to thank the UK regional directors of general practice and their associate advisers for sharing with me information about their hospital training courses. I would also like to express my special thanks to my regional director, Bob Berrington, and my fellow associate advisers, Simon Bailey, Arthur Hibble and Steve Lazar, for their support.

References

Academy of Royal Colleges (1997) *Recommendations for Training of Senior House Officers*. Academy of Royal Colleges, London.

Baker, M. (1993) Enhancing the educational content of SHO posts. *British Medical Journal* **306**, 808–809.

Bunch, G.A., Bahrami, J. & MacDonald, R. (1997) Training in the SHO grade. *British Journal of Hospital Medicine* **57**, 565–568.

Crawley, H.S. & Levin, J.B. (1990) Training for general practice: a national survey. *British Medical Journal* **300**, 911–915.

Firth-Cozens, J. (1987) Emotional distress in junior house officers. *British Medical Journal* **295**, 284–285.

General Medical Council, Education Subcommittee (1997) *The New Doctor*. GMC, London.

Grant, G. & Marsden, P. (1989) The plight of senior house officers—some facts. *Postgraduate Medical Journal* **65**, 869–871.

Hand, C.H. (1994) Joint hospital visiting: problems and solutions. *Postgraduate Education for General Practice* **5**, 247–253.

Hand, C.H. & Adams, M. (1998) The development and reliability of the Royal College of General Practitioners' questionnaire for measuring senior house officers' satisfaction with their hospital training. *British Journal of General Practice* **48**, 1399–1403.

Kelly, D.R. & Murray, T.S. (1991) Twenty years of vocational training in the west of Scotland. *British Medical Journal* **302**, 28–30.

Kelly, D. & Murray, T.S. (1997) An assessment of hospital training for general practice in Scotland. *Education for General Practice* **8**, 220–226.

Little, P. (1994) What do Wessex general practitioners think about the structure of hospital vocational training? *British Medical Journal* **308**, 1337–1339.

Moore, J.K., Neithercut, W.D., Mellors, A.S. *et al.* (1994) Making the new deal for junior doctors happen. *British Medical Journal* **308**, 1553–1555.

NHS Management Executive (1991) *The New Deal: Hours of Work of Doctors in Training*. Department of Health, London.

Paice, E., Moss, F., West, G. & Grant, J. (1997a) Association of a log book and experience as a preregistration house officer: interview survey. *British Medical Journal* **314**, 213–216.

Paice, E., West, G., Cooper, R., Orton, V. & Scotland, A. (1997b) Senior house officer training: is it getting better? *British Medical Journal* **314**, 719–720.

Pereira Gray, D. (1992) *Forty Years On—The Story of the First Forty Years of the Royal College of General Practitioners*. Royal College of General Practitioners, London.

Pringle, M., Hasler, J. & DeMarco, P. (1991) Training for minor surgery in general practice during preregistration Surgical Posts. *British Medical Journal* **302**, 830–832.

Reeve, H. & Bowman, A. (1989) Hospital training for general practice: views of trainees in the North Western region. *British Medical Journal* **298**, 1432–1434.

Royal College of General Practitioners (1994) *Education and Training for General Practice*. Policy Statement 3. RCGP, London.

Smith, A.G. & Cummings, C. (1997) Producing a guide to house jobs. *British Medical Journal* (classified supplement), 9 August.

Further reading

Hargreaves, D.H., Bowditch, M.G. & Griffin, D.R. (1997) *On-the-job Training for Surgeons.* Royal Society of Medicine Press, London.

Hargreaves, D.H., Southworth, G.W., Stanley, P. & Ward, S.J. (1997) *On-the-job Training for Physicians.* Royal Society of Medicine Press, London.

Joint Committee on Postgraduate Training for General Practice (1995) *Posts in Hospital and Public Health Medicine: General Guidance.* JCPTGP, London.

Joint Committee on Postgraduate Training for General Practice (1998) *A Guide to Certification.* JCPTGP, London.

Royal College of General Practitioners and Association for Palliative Medicine (1997) *Palliative Medicine Content of Vocational Training for General Practice.* RCGP, London.

Royal College of General Practitioners and British Association of Accident and Emergency Medicine (1997) *General Practitioner Vocational Training in Accident and Emergency Medicine.* RCGP, London.

Royal College of General Practitioners and British Geriatrics Society (1997) *General Practitioner Vocational Training in Geriatric Medicine.* RCGP, London.

Royal College of General Practitioners and Royal College of Obstetricians and Gynaecologists (1997) *General Practitioner Vocational Training in Obstetrics and Gynaecology.* RCGP, London.

Royal College of General Practitioners and Royal College of Paediatrics (1997) *The Paediatric Component of Vocational Training for General Practice.* RCGP, London.

Royal College of General Practitioners and Royal College of Psychiatrists (1997) *General Practitioner Vocational Training in Psychiatry.* RCGP, London.

3 Practice experience

Can there be learning without teaching? We know there can be teaching without learning.

[McEvoy, 1997]

Learning from the practice

For GP registrars, the training practice provides an astonishing wealth of learning opportunities. They have the privilege of being the only pupil of an experienced doctor who is also a trained teacher. In addition, they are able to enter and participate in a dynamic system of interacting professionals and patients. They join the practice rather like a social anthropologist carrying out a field study on an unknown culture. They are accepted by the indigenous people as one of their own; with the guidance of their trainer, they learn their skills. Registrars are able to observe the customs and rituals of the practice with an objective eye; to see what works well and what does not work well; to reflect on how things might be done differently.

The first week

It is important for the registrar to feel welcome and to be recognized by the practice (Samuel, 1990).

Preparations should be made for the registrar's arrival (see Box 3.1) and introduction to the partners, the practice manager and all the primary care team members. Everyone should know who and what the new doctor is. Great efforts should be made to provide the registrar with a room of his or her own with a nameplate on the door. If this is not possible, the registrar should be able to use the same room each day and have sufficient space for books, equipment and personal effects.

Box 3.1 Preparing for the new registrar

• Room cleared of debris left by previous occupant and cleaned
• Good supply of all necessary stationery
• Computer installed and running and password supplied
• Name on the door
• Staff informed
• Patients informed (e.g. by notice at reception)
• Pay and deductions worked out by manager
• Duty rota agreed
• Library tidied and contents reviewed
• Educational contract signed

The educational contract

In addition to the normal contract of employment, it is helpful for the trainer and registrar to agree and sign an educational contract. This sets out the contribution which each will make towards the registrar's education in general practice. The items covered will usually include hours of attendance for surgeries and visits, on-call commitments, entitlement to annual leave and study leave, timing of tutorials and other protected teaching times. If these matters are all agreed at the beginning, there are unlikely to be subsequent disagreements or misunderstandings about how much work and how much teaching are expected.

The induction period

Trainer and registrar will draw up between them a timetable for the induction period (usually about 2 weeks). In this period the registrar will learn something about the consultation process and the clinical scope of general practice by sitting in with the trainer during surgery sessions. The registrar will also spend time with the other partners and team members, observing what they do and trying to make sense of it. An example of a timetable is given in Box 3.2.

Box 3.2 First week: example of a timetable

Monday	a.m.: surgery and visits with trainer
	p.m.: orientation tutorial; surgery with trainer
Tuesday	a.m.: observe receptionist (and be a receptionist), talk to manager
	p.m.: paediatric clinic; meet practice nurse and health visitor
Wednesday	a.m.: surgery with another partner
	p.m.: with health visitor
Thursday	a.m.: surgery and visits with trainer
	p.m.: with practice nurse
Friday	a.m.: surgery with third partner; practice meeting
	free time

Box 3.3 Inner team

Business partners, employees of the practice, attached colleagues from other disciplines:
• Doctors (partners, assistants, other GP registrars)
• Manager
• Receptionists and secretaries
• Practice nurses
• District nurses
• Community psychiatric nurse
• Health visitor
• Midwives
• Counsellors
• Other 'in-house' therapists: e.g. physiotherapist, osteopath

---

Meeting the team(s)

During the first few weeks the registrar will be able to meet and spend time with a large number of people—those in the 'inner team' (see Box 3.3), who work closely with the doctors, and others in the 'outer team' (see Box 3.4), who are more loosely associated with the practice but equally important.

Box 3.4 Outer team

- Independent or health or local authority-based colleagues
- Pharmacist
- Palliative care nurse
- Chiropodist
- Dietician
- Social workers
- Optometrist

Box 3.5 Worksheet for sitting in with a partner

- How does his/her style differ from your trainer's?
- Does he/she see a different group of patients?
- Is he/she a tight timekeeper?
- Is he/she a high or low prescriber?
- How readily does he/she refer patients?
- Is he/she involved and empathic or cool and distant?
- Is he/she enthusiastic about health promotion?

Getting the best out of 'sitting in'

A registrar will gain more satisfaction and learn more from a sitting-in session if some sort of guide or template is supplied, around which his or her observations can be structured and curiosity stimulated. Help will be needed in formulating some good questions to ask the person being observed and to encourage self-questioning. The trainer can assist by providing a 'worksheet' with a few sample questions (see Boxes 3.5 & 3.6).

The answers to these questions (and others generated by the registrar) can form the basis for a discussion of the experience at a subsequent tutorial. In this way the registrar is likely to reflect more and to learn more than if the trainer merely asks 'how did you get on with the health visitor?'—to which the answer may just be: 'fine, thanks'.

Similar worksheets can be designed by the trainer (and the registrar) for use in sessions with all the other team members.

> **Box 3.6** Worksheet for observing the health visitor
> - What does a health visitor do?
> - What are their statutory duties?
> - Who is their manager and employer? (Compare with practice nurse)
> - How much are health visitors paid? (Compare with doctors)
> - What do they like best about the job?
> - What do they find frustrating?
> - How do their working styles differ from that of a practice nurse or a social worker?

Needs assessment: where are we starting from?

Some time in the first week, perhaps at the first tutorial, registrar and trainer will sit down together and discuss the registrar's learning needs so that they can begin to draw up a curriculum.

They might begin by looking at the registrar's experience so far: the posts held and the clinical skills acquired. Then they might consider the registrar's current view of general practice and his or her current thinking about the discipline. The trainer will then offer a picture of the GP's role, responsibilities and work content. The registrar can review his or her clinical knowledge with the help of a syllabus checklist, ticking the appropriate column in a confidence rating scale. A simple MCQ test will help to assess the registrar's factual knowledge base. Enlightened by all this information and reflection, the registrar and trainer together can draw up a learning plan for the first few months. At the end of this first teaching term they will review their achievements and the registrar's new position on the learning curve can be plotted. This formative assessment (see Box 3.7) enables them to discover the registrar's current learning needs and to plan the next term's work.

Teaching occasions, style and methods

There are many occasions in the life of the teaching practice when learning can take place, either formally or informally. One of the

---

Box 3.7 Initial needs assessment

- Summary of registrar's experience so far: posts held and clinical skills acquired
- View of general practice: what is it about? (Trainer's view; registrar's view)
- The GP's area of responsibilities and work content (presented by trainer)
- MCQs to check registrar's clinical knowledge
- Registrar's own assessment of strengths and weaknesses
- Checklist of skills and confidence ratings

Box 3.8 Teaching occasions

- Tutorials
- Joint surgeries and visits
- Out-of-hours co-operative sessions
- Daily debriefing (after surgery)
- Requests for help during or after surgery (difficult cases)
- Observing colleagues (with worksheet)
- Teaching sessions with colleagues
- Investigating practice systems (see Box 3.13)
- Practice meetings
- Team meeting; partners' meeting; clinical meeting; journal club

---

trainer's important skills is the ability to turn everyday events into learning opportunities.

Box 3.8 provides some examples of occasions that can be turned into learning opportunities.

Teaching style

Trainers will have different personalities, which will influence their styles and the way they relate to their registrars. Nevertheless, we can identify some important qualities and techniques which all good trainers have in common:

Being a good listener. The trainer should be accessible and approachable. He or she should not mind having surgery interrupted if the registrar has a problem. In case discussions, the trainer will make the registrar feel that full attention and empathic concern is being given. This approach also models the way a doctor listens to a patient and will help the registrar to listen helpfully to his or her own patients.

Assessing while listening. Assessment is a continuous process, and every time the registrar talks about work the trainer has an opportunity silently to check out the registrar's knowledge of the subject being discussed, attitude to the patient and emotional state.

Reflecting the question. Many informal teaching encounters will begin with a question from the registrar. If the trainer answers by providing information (e.g. the likely diagnosis, the best prescription, the recommended referral), the immediate problem will be solved but the registrar will not have been given an opportunity to think for him or herself.

'Reflecting the question' means inviting the registrar to make use of what is already known and to come up with a plan of action. It should not be done mechanically; for example, by asking the question 'What do **you** think you should do?' A better phrase might be 'let's think what the options might be here'. They might be ordering some blood tests, writing a prescription, telephoning a consultant for advice or referral to hospital. The likely consequences of each alternative can then be discussed so that the registrar can make a decision. The trainer may be able to recommend some relevant reading and the outcome can be discussed at a later date. All this takes time and there are occasions, perhaps when the registrar is under a lot of stress, when it might be better just to give advice and discuss the question more fully later on.

Providing resources. The trainer can help the registrar to be responsible for self learning by recommending sources of information rather than giving a lecture (see Box 3.9).

Widening the view in case discussion. Discussion of individual cases is of central importance in learning general practice.

The trainer can help the registrar to avoid too narrow a view of the patient's problem. GP training pioneered the concept of

---

Box 3.9 Sources of information

- Books in the library
- Journal articles
- Trainer's file of useful articles
- Patient records
- Computer searches
- Searching Medline via the Internet
- Accessing CD ROM information
- Talking to consultants and other specialists
- Talking to patients

Box 3.10 Issues arising from a case

1 What did the patient want?
2 What were the patient's own thoughts and feelings about the problem?
3 Did the doctor have a different agenda?
4 Did they agree on a diagnosis and plan?
5 What family and psychosocial issues might have been significant?
6 Were there any practice management issues?
7 How did the doctor feel about the consultation?

'diagnosis in multiple dimensions'. These were originally three dimensions: physical, psychological and social (Royal College of General Practitioners, 1972). Problems in the practice and its systems, which may come to light when a case is considered in depth, also need to be diagnosed. Learning from case discussion is enriched if trainer and registrar consider some of the issues arising as well as the immediate diagnosis and management of the patient's problem (see Box 3.10).

Example: A 5-year-old with a sore throat
1 The mother wanted a prescription for an antibiotic.
2 She was afraid her child might get worse otherwise.
3 The doctor wanted to use paracetamol only.
4 They agreed to start with paracetamol and review after 2 days.

5 The doctor saw from the notes that the mother was unsupported and had a history of postnatal depression.

6 The mother mentioned that she had had difficulty in getting an appointment.

7 The registrar felt that the mother had been angry at first, but then became more willing to trust the registrar after time had been spent examining the child and explaining the reasoning.

Note: Any of these issues could be listed for further research and discussion.

The trainer has an opportunity to make an assessment of the registrar's awareness of the issues and ability to deal with them. This assessment can be recorded in an assessment log or diary and subsequently discussed with the registrar. The registrar can learn more about some of the issues (e.g. postnatal depression) and demonstrate his or her increased capability at a later assessment.

Other ways of learning about the consultation

Video recording

This is a uniquely valuable way for the registrar to see and hear exactly what happens in consultations. Video recording has now become a regular feature, rather than an occasional novelty, as a result of the need to provide tapes for summative assessment and the MRCGP examination.

The practice needs to acquire a suitable camcorder. It is probably better for the registrar to learn to use the camcorder and to edit the tapes, so that recording sessions can be planned and looked at in privacy. The tapes can then be discussed with the trainer. The original guidelines for reviewing tapes were provided by Pendleton *et al.* (1984). A more recent approach (Silverman *et al.*, 1998a,b) suggests that it is useful for the registrar to say what it was he or she hoped to achieve in the consultation and in which areas help was needed.

Looking at a video enables the registrar to observe the consultation style and, perhaps, to consider ways in which it might be modified. It is a good idea for trainers to show registrars their own recordings of consultations at an early stage, to demonstrate that they are not afraid to expose themselves to scrutiny. If there are a few mistakes, so much the better.

Registrars (and trainers) will particularly notice obvious problems with consultation style, such as:

- Preoccupation with rummaging through notes or staring at the computer screen instead of concentrating on the patient.
- Talking too much and asking too many closed questions.
- Irritating mannerisms.

When problems of this sort have been recognized and solved by a change of style, the registrar and trainer can look at some of the more subtle aspects of the art of consultation. As they view a taped consultation, they will ask themselves:

- Does the doctor notice evidence of the patient's feelings? (the depressive posture, the break in the voice, the clenched fist, the finger brushing away an unshed tear).
- Does the doctor pick up verbal cues about the patient's preoccupations?, e.g. When the patient says: 'I thought it might be my heart', does the doctor say: 'No, it isn't' or 'what made you think it might be your heart?'.
- Do doctor and patient listen to each other and agree on a plan of action?
- What was the doctor trying to achieve and how far was this successful?
- Did the patient seem satisfied that he or she had been properly heard?

On a more basic clinical level, the trainer and registrar can check that the appropriate examination, investigation and referral are being done and that an obvious diagnosis has not been missed.

Looking at the video is not simply an exercise in spotting mistakes. The trainer and registrar may take considerable satisfaction from observing sensitive and constructive consultations. If all goes well, the trainer will note with pleasure the pupil's progress in acquiring and refining skills.

Joint consultations

In the first few weeks the registrar will learn a great deal about general practice just from sitting with the trainer. The initial picture of what a GP is like will reflect the trainer's approach and style, and the view of the right way to consult may continue to be strongly influenced by those first impressions. There will be opportunities to compare and contrast the trainer with other doctors and the registrar will also develop a personal style as time goes on. Nevertheless, the trainer will always be an important model. The trainer therefore needs to set a good example, hopefully one in which the doctor is not overinvolved with work and patients and has time to relax and be with family or pursue other interests beyond general practice!

When the registrar has gained a little more experience and is used to carrying out consultations alone, the joint surgery can be used for a joint approach, with both doctors contributing to the discussion with and about the patient. At this stage, the registrar can look more objectively at the trainer's approach, and decide which elements of the trainer's technique to incorporate into his or her work and which to discard. The trainer can now observe the registrar at work directly and incorporate this in the registrar's continuous formative assessment process.

Are you seeing the right patients?

Unless there is positive intervention by the trainer, there will be significant differences between the patients appearing on the trainer's surgery list and those the registrar sees (compare Boxes 3.11 & 3.12). Principal GPs acquire a faithful following of regular patients after a few years and are more likely to see those with chronic illnesses. Registrars tend to see those who book appointments at the last minute or ask to be seen as 'emergencies'.

The unplanned registrar's list provides a wealth of excitement and experience. However, as time goes on, the registrar will need to see more of the kind of patients seen by the trainer in order to broaden the range. Trainer and registrar can compare lists and review the gaps in the registrar's clinical experience every few months. The registrar can be introduced to some patients with chronic diseases and encouraged to follow them up. It is important for the registrar to develop long-term relationships with some patients and their families for the duration of the attachment to the practice.

Box 3.11 A typical trainer's list

- Elderly hypertensive
- Diabetic patient
- Woman with complicated gynaecological history
- Elderly patient who has grown old with the doctor
- Patient with multiple chronic diseases
- Patient with terminal illness
- Bereavement
- Marital problem
- Chronic neurological problem (MS, Parkinsonism)
- Ischaemic heart disease

Box 3.12 A typical registrar's list

- Small child with feverish illness
- Contraceptive advice
- Minor injuries
- Acute asthma attack
- 'Heartsink' patient seeking a new home
- Drug and alcohol problems
- People wanting certificates and letters
- Temporary residents
- Low back strain
- Panic attacks

The content of general practice: what should a registrar learn?

The trainer and the registrar come to each other with different perspectives on general practice, which need to be shared. The registrar brings hospital experience, which will powerfully influence expectations; the registrar will probably expect to see much serious disease and may be disappointed that there is so little in general practice. They may feel that hard-won skills are in danger of rusting. On the other hand, some of the demands which the patients make (letters, certificates, attention to their point of view) may make them feel inappropriately used or even abused.

The trainer, on the other hand, is familiar with the reality of general practice, although striving to change it. He or she may have a vision of what general practice is about and this needs to be shared with the registrar. Alternative visions will be available from other team members, from books and articles and from the discussions at the release course.

One way to survey the territory is to draw up a list of the GP's activities, necessary skills and responsibilities. The trainer and registrar can consult the list at intervals, add to it where appropriate and fill in the gaps in the registrar's knowledge and experience. The syllabus below represents only one version:

A syllabus for general practice

The syllabus outlined here will then be discussed in more detail under the appropriate headings:

1 Diagnosis and care of acute illness.
2 Management of chronic illness.
3 Psychosocial problems.
4 Preventive medicine and health education.
5 Practice management.
6 Professional and personal development.

1. Acute illness

The doctor needs to be able to:
• Listen attentively and enable patient to reveal themselves.
• Recognize all of the common illnesses and many less common ones.
• Employ clinical reasoning in the more difficult diagnoses.
• Agree a plan of management.
• Practice evidence-based medicine.
• Prescribe effectively and economically.
• Deal with emergencies.
• Request appropriate investigations.
• Refer to colleagues appropriately and write a good letter.
• Explain procedures, treatment and prognosis to the patient.

2. Chronic illness (examples: arthritis, diabetes, multiple sclerosis, elderly patients with multiple pathology, terminal illness)

The doctor needs to be able to:

- Make an assessment of the nature and severity of the disability.
- Review and revise medication.
- Enlist help from colleagues in primary and secondary care.
- Arrange social and ancillary services.
- Co-ordinate efforts of team members.
- Provide personal and continuing care.
- Set up chronic disease management systems.
- Audit quality and standards.

3. Psychosocial problems (examples: marital problems, substance abuse, clinical depression, personal unhappiness)

The doctor should be able to:
- Be receptive to any request for help.
- Use the medical model where appropriate.
- Enlist help from other professionals (counsellor, community psychiatric nurse, social worker).
- Provide time to listen.
- Utilize counselling skills.
- Consider family and systemic aspects.
- Follow up patients personally.
- Learn to cope with powerful emotions in self and patients.
- Balance empathy with objectivity.

Note: The many psychosomatic illnesses encountered in general practice require a combination of the skills in 1, 2 and 3.

4. Preventive medicine and health education

The doctor should be able to organize preventive services, for example:
- Well-baby clinic.
- Surveillance of the elderly.
- Immunization for children and adults at risk.
- Screening and case finding for chronic diseases, e.g. diabetes, hypertension.
- Cervical cytology.
- Cardiovascular risk factor management, e.g. smoking, diet, exercise, alcohol.

5. Practice management

The doctor should be able to provide and maintain systems which enable patients to reach and benefit from practice services easily:
• Appointment systems.
• On-call and out-of-hours arrangements.
• Repeat prescriptions.
  The doctor should know about:
• Design, purchase and maintenance of premises.
• Staff training and management.
• Records (manual and electronic).
• Financial matters.
• The role of the practice manager.
• Planning and introducing changes.
• Primary Care Groups.

6. Professional and personal development

The doctor should:
• Have a personal continuing education plan.
• Cultivate the habit of regularly reading books and journal articles relevant to general practice.
• Audit practice systems and clinical activities to ensure that standards are set and maintained.
• Keep up to date with information technology.
• Make use of the best clinical evidence available.
• Be sufficiently curious to become involved in some research activity.
• Avoid an excessive workload.
• Have outside interests.
• Have time for family and friends.
• Share problems and seek personal help when needed.

Investigating the practice and its systems

The practice will have a number of continuing activities, the smooth running of which is regulated by a system. The registrar will learn more about practice systems by investigating them personally than by listening to the trainer talking about them (see Box 3.13).

Box 3.13 Practice systems

- Repeat prescribing
- Appointments
- Patient–staff relationships
- Staff management
- Cervical cytology
- Out-of-hours care
- Emergencies
- Dealing with deaths
- Record keeping
- Routine visits
- Complaints
- Practice meetings
- Maintenance of premises

Ideas for investigations may arise from clinical situations, for example:
- Why do we prescribe so much ranitidine?
- How do diabetics get their eyes checked?
- Who gets regular visits and why?
- Could a death have been prevented?

Example: What's wrong with the appointment system?
The registrar is concerned that patients are complaining that they find it difficult to book appointments and asks if the trainer thinks there is a problem, suggesting an investigation of the current working of the system. They discuss how this is to be done.

They decide that the registrar will:
1 Discuss the appointment system with the manager.
2 Look at the number of emergency appointments available each week.
3 Observe a receptionist making appointments.
4 Record the time to the earliest routine appointment offered to a consecutive series of patients.
5 Find out how receptionists deal with patients who 'must be seen today'.

The appointment system might also be compared with that in a neighbouring practice.

The registrar's findings can be discussed at a subsequent tutorial. The findings can be used as the basis of an audit. Any recommendations for improvement can then be presented at a practice meeting. This will be another useful learning opportunity.

The advantages of the method are summarized below:
- The registrar has learned actively instead of listening passively.
- The registrar has learned something about how to plan and carry out an operational research project.
- The registrar now has some practical knowledge of an important aspect of practice administration which will be invaluable when he or she becomes a principal.

Example: How to stay awake at practice meetings
It is usually recommended that registrars attend practice meetings. Often they find meetings boring because:
- Their own concerns are not involved (e.g. money, hours of work, responsibilities, dealing with change).
- They have no knowledge of the dynamics of meetings.
- They have not read anything about modern management theory.

The registrar will find the meeting much more interesting and enjoyable if he or she is prepared.

The trainer might suggest:
- Reading a few chapters in a management book, concentrating on such themes as 'bringing about change', 'chairing a meeting' and 'how to get what you want out of a meeting'.
- Finding out how the manager would like to see the practice developing.

During the meeting, taking special note of:
- The quality of chairing.
- The different roles of the participants.
- Who is getting what they want.
- Who is not being heard.
- Alliances and conflicts.

Afterwards the registrar can report the findings to the trainer and they can compare their perceptions.

Reading and the practice library

The teaching practice should pride itself on the quality of its library. Everyone should be invited to contribute suggestions about books to buy and one partner (probably the trainer but not necessarily) can be responsible for buying books and keeping the library up to date.

The library should include:

- A few good reference books on all relevant subjects (ear, nose and throat, ophthalmology, dermatology, clinical anatomy, surgery, neurology).
- Clinical specialty textbooks written from a general practice perspective, for example:
  Womens' Problems in General Practice by Ann McPherson
  Efficient Care in General Practice by Geoffrey Marsh
  Paediatric Problems in General Practice by Michael Modell and Robert Boyd.
  Providing Diabetes Care in General Practice by Mary MacKinnon
- Classic books about general practice, for example:
  The Doctor, his Patient and the Illness by Michael Balint
  A Fortunate Man by John Berger
  Epidemiology in Country Practice by William Pickles
  Doctor Talking to Patients by Patrick Byrne and Barrie Long
  The Inner Consultation by Roger Neighbour
  Culture, Health and Illness by Cecil Helman.
- Books about research, epidemiology and evidence-based medicine, for example:
  Research in General Practice by C. Howie.
- Books about management and the business of general practice.
- Books about medicine and society, for example:
  Limits to Medicine by Ivan Illch
  Inequalities in Health: The Black Report by Peter Townsend and Mick Davidson.
- Books dealing with the wider field of interpersonal relationships, including:
- Counselling and psychotherapy.
- Books dealing with medical ethics.
- Books dealing with death and bereavement, for example:
  Bereavement by Colin Murray Parkes
  Death and Dying by Elisabeth Kubler Ross.

- General books containing observations of people and their lives, for example:
  The People of Providence by Tony Parker.
- Some classic novels, with or without doctors as characters:
  Anna Karenina by Leo Tolstoy
  Metamorphosis, A Country Doctor and other stories by Franz Kafka
  Middlemarch by George Eliot
  The Mayor of Casterbridge by Thomas Hardy
  Madam Bovary by Gustave Flaubert.

The trainer and registrar may enjoy comparing notes on the books each is reading during the course of the year (Samuel, 1990).

The library will also contain copies of a few relevant journals going back for about 3–5 years. Suggested journals are:

- *The British Journal of General Practice.*
- *The British Medical Journal.*
- *Education for General Practice.*
- *The Prescribers' Journal.*

The RCGP's series of Occasional Papers is also well worth collecting.

Formative assessment

Assessment is a continuous process:
- It needs to be shared to make it formative.
- It should always include the registrar's self assessment.

Discussion of consultations

All contacts between trainer and registrar provide material for assessing the registrar's progress. Information is gathered from:
- joint consultations and visits
- observation of clinical skills (e.g. speculum examination)
- tutorials
- discussions about projects
- feedback on practice system studies
- videos
- audits

- formal tests (see below).
  Information is also gathered from others in the practice:
- partners
- nurses and health visitors
- receptionists
- patients.

The assessment diary

An **assessment diary** is a useful way to make sure that the assessment keeps rolling. The trainer keeps notes of the registrar's progress in all areas of general practice learning. The trainer will note the acquisition of a new skill (e.g. tennis elbow injection) and an improvement in consultation style (using more open questions). The trainer may note the need to learn a skill (perhaps ear syringing) or to find out more information (e.g. the pharmacological treatment of hypertension).

The diary needs to be shared regularly with the registrar so that plans can be agreed for filling in gaps in knowledge and finding opportunities to learn or improve skills.

An example of a diary entry after a tutorial on diabetes is given below:

'Good general knowledge about the physiology, complications, diagnosis and treatment. Why do we think it is important to control blood sugar and blood pressure? Look up evidence that good control can reduce complications. Learn more about management in general practice by sitting in with practice nurse at her diabetic clinic. Arrange to attend hospital clinic to see some diabetic eye signs.'

A subsequent entry (in a parallel column) can record a reassessment after the proposed work has been carried out, for example:

'Has been to eye clinic and now more confident about viewing dilated fundus and detecting diabetic retinopathy.'

Formal assessments

These are helpful if carried out serially, but not too often. The modules of summative assessment (MCQs, audit, video) are usually carried out well before the end of the training period and can take their place as formative assessments.

Multiple choice test. This is useful to check basic clinical knowledge. Weak spots can be identified in order to focus reading where it is needed.

Modified essay questions. These questions will demonstrate the registrar's ability to think laterally and be aware of all the issues arising from a clinical situation. Books of questions are available but it is more fun to make up your own or base them on real events in the practice.

Rating scales (e.g. Rating Scales for Vocational Training in General Practice, Centre for Primary Care Research, 1988). These are time-consuming and indigestible if swallowed whole. A better way is to use a few scales only and allow them to generate points for discussion.

Examples from 'Manchester' Scales (Centre for Primary Care Research, 1988):
- Scale 11 (Management 1: coping with uncertainty): discuss examples of ongoing cases where diagnosis is still uncertain.
- Scale 15 (Medical records): show each other examples of records and discuss their quality.
- Scale 21 (Professionalism 3: communication): discuss encounters with angry, distressed or flirtatious patients.

Clinical skills

Basic clinical skills are supposed to be learned in medical school training and hospital posts. In reality, some registrars will not have acquired sufficient ability or confidence in some procedures. The training practice provides the opportunity to make good these deficiencies. In addition, there are other skills derived from hospital specialties in which the registrar never worked and which are now part of general practice. These include the skills necessary to deal with emergencies.

The trainer and registrar can check the registrar's 'confidence rating' in each procedure. The registrar's level of skill with patients can be assessed by the trainer, or someone else: a partner or a nurse, who can provide feedback for the trainer and registrar. Further experience and teaching can then be arranged where appropriate.

Basic skills

- Dealing with emergencies (haemorrhage, acute asthma, myocardial infarction).
- General physical examination of all systems.
- Vaginal examination and cervical screening.
- Rectal examination and, perhaps, proctoscopy.
- Musculoskeletal system (back, knees, shoulders), which has often been inadequately taught.
- Use of ophthalmoscope and auriscope.
- Blood taking.
- Cardiopulmonary resuscitation.
- Intramuscular injections.

GP skills

- Ear syringing.
- Joint and soft tissue injection.
- Use of peak-flow meter.
- Nebulizer.
- ECG.
- Minor surgery procedures.
- Examination of infants.
- Psychiatric emergencies.

Outside attachments

Registrars often feel the need to learn more about certain specialties which commonly occur in the surgery and seem to perplex trainer and registrar equally. Freshly released from a hospital environment, the registrar may feel that the only way to become competent in ear, nose and throat or dermatology is to return to the hospital and 'sit at the feet of a consultant'.

Trainers are frequently asked to arrange, or at least agree to, short-term attachments to clinics such as ear, nose and throat, dermatology, ophthalmology, rheumatology or genitourinary medicine. It is difficult to know whether these attachments are really worthwhile. Clinical knowledge and skills are more likely to result from doing and taking responsibility rather than sitting and watching. Outreach clinics, where the hospital clinic visits the practice to advise on the practice's patients, are likely to provide better learning opportunities. If the registrar does attend a hospital clinic, a list of objectives should be taken which have been drawn up in discussion with the trainer.

Some examples of these objectives are:
- Ophthalmology clinic: learn to recognize common signs of diabetic retinopathy.
- Rheumatology clinic: learn to inject a tennis elbow and a rotator cuff (shoulder) lesion.

Why not visit another practice?

Registrars who have done this often remember it as one of the most formative experiences of their GP training. It is best to arrange an exchange of registrars with a contrasting practice. A country practice will clearly provide a very different experience from that in an inner-city area; however, dramatic contrasts can be found within a city between practices with different populations or different philosophies. The registrar who has become used to highly educated and sophisticated professionals as patients will have much to think about after a fortnight trying to deal with people who are desperately poor, inadequately housed and perhaps recently arrived from non-English-speaking countries.

The registrar will come back from the attachment to a contrasting practice with a new vantage point from which to see general practice as a whole. He or she will have new ideas to try out in the home practice and a new appreciation of some of the things in the home practice which now appear, on reflection, to work quite well. To the trainer, the registrar may suddenly seem much more mature.

References

Centre for Primary Care Research, Department of General Practice, University of Manchester (1988) *Rating Scales for Vocational Training in General Practice*. Royal College of General Practitioners, London.

McEvoy, P. (1997) Personal communication. Ripon, Yorkshire.

Pendleton, D., Schofield, T., Tate, P. & Havelock, P. (1984) *The Consultation. An Approach to Learning and Teaching.* Oxford University Press, Oxford.

Royal College of General Practitioners (1972) *The Future General Practitioner—Learning and Teaching.* BMJ Publishing Group, London.

Samuel, O. (1990) *Towards a Curriculum for General Practice.* Occasional Paper 44. Royal College of General Practitioners, London.

Silverman, J., Kurtz, S. & Draper, J. (1998a) *Teaching and Learning Communication Skills in Medicine.* Radcliffe Medical Press, Abingdon, UK.

Silverman, J., Kurtz, S. & Draper, J. (1998b) *Skills for Communicating with Patients.* Radcliffe Medical Press, Abingdon, UK.

4 The one-to-one tutorial

Introduction

The one-to-one tutorial is at the heart of training. In the quiet of the tutorial session, the registrar and trainer can explore areas of difficulty, support and nurture each other and empower learning. To achieve this several things need to be in place:

1 The trainer needs to ensure protected time and a place free from interruption.

2 A learning environment that is sensitive to the registrar's needs.

3 The style of the tutorial should ideally be learner-centred, but it needs to be flexible, so that the agenda of both the registrar and the trainer can be met.

4 There must be evaluation of the tutorial, both its content and process, not only by the registrar, but also by the trainer.

5 Plans for future learning can be made on the basis of material that has been explored during the session.

Preparation

Tutorials need to be regular and the time allocated for them should be protected. Regions will have written standards detailing how often tutorials should take place. The minimum frequency will be weekly, lasting for at least one and a half hours, although more frequent and longer sessions are common. It is important that the tutorial takes place on the registrar's territory, where he or she will feel secure and more able to discuss sensitive issues.

Advance preparation is needed for every tutorial, but this does not necessarily mean extensive reading for the trainer. It is important, though, to reflect on the happenings of the week; for example, were there any events involving the registrar which need further exploration? What is also useful is to revisit notes made in previous tutorials. Are there topics that you agreed to cover that have not yet been looked at? Is the registrar avoiding certain subjects because they are contentious or because he or she is uncomfortable dealing with them?

Preparation also takes place through formative assessment, with the curriculum being planned in the early weeks of the registrar's attachment. This is dealt with in Chapter 3.

Content

As described later in this chapter under 'Self-directed learning', the content of the tutorials can be led by registrar need. There also needs to be space for the trainer's 'professional' agenda, helping the registrar look at areas that are difficult or uncomfortable to talk about. The Johari window can show how self-examination, together with feedback from the trainer, can help the registrar develop self-awareness (Fig. 4.1) (Luft & Harrington, 1984). The open area describes things that are known to the registrar and to others. The hidden part shows things about the registrar that are known only to him or her but not to others. Exploration of this area may help a registrar develop trust and confidence.

Others know the blind area but not the registrar. Positive feedback here can help the registrar become more self-aware. This will help in work with others. The dark, undiscovered area consists of feelings, conflicts, abilities and so on which the registrar is not aware of and which others have not seen. This area also contains problems, and investigating this area may prove extremely stressful for the registrar, and may need counselling or psychotherapy.

The Future General Practitioner—Learning and Teaching (Royal College of General Practitioners, 1972) categorizes broad areas of practice which are of great help in planning tutorials and in ensuring that no key area is omitted. The five areas are:

- Health and disease.
- Human development.
- Human behaviour.
- Medicine and society.
- Practice organization.

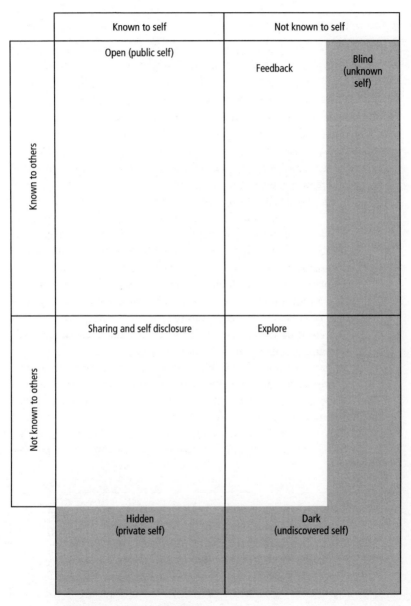

Figure 4.1 The Johari window.

Resources

The trainer does not have to teach every subject—there are plenty of people available within (and outside) the primary health care team who are able to teach in their professional area. The library too is an essential resource. However, to be useful the library needs to be relevant to general practice, and to be classified and ordered in a logical way. The Dewey system of classification is one way of doing this, in which there are 10 main classes of knowledge numbered 0 to 9. Useful arts are classified number 6, and medicine is subclass 61. Many libraries use the National Library of Medicine classification, which is designed specifically for a medical collection. Here clinical subjects are classed under the letter W, with the practice of medicine under letters WB. Your local librarian will be able to advise on the best method to use, or further reading can be found in Morton and Wright (1990). Even a simple system of cataloguing, using markers and keywords, can help a registrar get the most from the library. This can either be held electronically or on a card system.

Registrars are expected to have a critical understanding of GP-relevant literature, both books and journals. This requires the trainer to be up to date in his or her reading of GP literature. Help in critical appraisal may be obtained from a local research unit or academic department. The registrar will want to be able to search for relevant material using MEDLINE or an equivalent source (Box 4.1). Many practices now have on-line access to this via the British Medical Association Library, but the World Wide Web

---

Box 4.1 Some useful Web addresses

National Library of Medicine	http://www4.ncbi.nlm.nih.gov/ PubMed/
Bandolier	http://www.jr2.ox.ac.uk/Bandolier/ index.html
Royal College of GPs	http://www.rcgp.org.uk/college/ index/html
British Medical Journal	http://www.bmj.com/bmj/
South-west libraries site	http://www.soton.ac.uk/~swhclu/

also has easy access to much useful material. MEDLINE can be accessed free of charge through the National Library of Medicine site. Some other useful Web addresses are listed in Box 4.1.

Supervision

Supervision is the norm in many of the caring professions, but is rare in general practice. Supervision is a protective, restorative and monitoring process that enables the registrar to discuss problems and issues with a colleague. This is really the role of the tutorial, the place where the registrar can come to the trainer, who acts as manager, teacher, supporter and appraiser. This is a tough role for the trainer to take on, and he or she will also need supervision to enable them to work effectively. It is helpful to identify where that will come from—in many areas the trainers' workshops will be useful, in others a training colleague or partner may take on the role.

What makes a good supervisor? The person needs to be flexible and able to adjust to the needs of the registrar. They need to be attentive and curious, listening carefully to the words and nuances of the recipient. They need to be concerned and caring, with 'unconditional positive regard'. In summary, they have to be structured, thorough, affirming, supportive and sensitive (Kaye, personal communication, 1997).

It is difficult to be all these things to one person. It needs space and time, good communication and counselling skills, with a clear contract of what is expected through the tutorials—and through training in general. The trainer and registrar both need to be aware of the boundaries of this relationship. They need to decide how close a friendship can be allowed to develop, and they both need to know where to seek help and advice should the relationship go wrong. Usually help can be sought from the local course organizers, or if necessary from the director of postgraduate education.

Learning styles

Kolb and Fry (1975) were among the first authors to describe a model of experiential learning, building on the work of Dewey,

Lewin and Piaget. They described four stages of learning—
experiencing, reflecting, concluding and testing. Honey and
Mumford (1986) developed this into learning styles. They postu-
lated that learners have four characteristic styles: activist, reflector,
theorist and pragmatist.

The activist likes to do, to try anything once. They learn best
from exposure to challenges, learning least well from passive
'lecture-style' presentations. Problem-based learning may work
best for them.

Reflectors, on the other hand, like to feel, and need time to get
into a new situation. They need space and time to ponder experiences and to absorb new information before making a considered
judgement. They need time to plan, and find it difficult coping
with the spontaneous tutorial.

Theorists are most comfortable with activities that enable them
to integrate experience into logically constructed theories and
models. They like to think and to see how things fit together.
They will not be happy with superficial answers and will probe
ever deeper for solutions to their problems.

The pragmatist likes to decide, and wants to know how a new
experience can be applied in practice. They prefer activities that
have a clear practical value, and when they can test out their ideas
in a real situation. This means that learning needs to have clear
applicability.

Although we all have our preferred style, this does not
mean that we cannot learn in any other style. All parts of the
cycle are needed for a good learning experience. It is important
to remember that we tend to start the cycle in our dominant
style, so it is worth considering the registrar's style and how this
can be most effectively linked to the learning process. We also
tend to teach in our main learning style, so an activist trainer
loves to do and experience, but this can be very difficult for the
reflector registrar to comprehend. This mismatch in styles can
be so extreme that training fails. It is also useful to remember
that an extreme in one learning style can be both a benefit and
a handicap.

Learning-style questionnaires can be obtained direct from
Honey and Mumford (at Peter Honey, Ardingly House, 10 Linden
Avenue, Maidenhead, Berks SL6 6HB), although the vocational

training scheme may introduce these to registrars early in their attachment year (Honey & Mumford, 1986).

Teaching styles

We tend to teach in four basic styles. All styles are useful for helping the registrar to learn particular aspects of general practice. The first style, the didactic, is characterized by the passing of information or facts with little intellectual processing by the registrar. This style may be useful at the beginning of training, or when new information has to be passed quickly, but if used on its own it does not encourage retention or understanding.

The Socratic style describes a carefully planned series of questions asked in order to lead the registrar towards a deeper understanding of a particular problem. This method is useful in developing understanding but it does not necessarily help analysis and evaluation. It is certainly more useful if the questions are open rather than closed, and the registrar is encouraged to develop insight and active participation.

Counselling, with its open questions, summarizing and reflection, is the most appropriate style when the registrar is becoming more experienced and needing less direction and support. It is invaluable for helping a registrar explore topics and areas that are difficult.

A registrar is ready for the heuristic approach when they need no direction and minimal support. Here the registrar is feeling confident and is already competent. Work is delegated to the registrar and he or she will work well alone. However, it is important to remember that this is not equivalent to abdication of responsibility for helping the registrar. He or she will still need feedback, and new areas of work will need a style that is appropriate to their level of knowledge and skills.

These styles are not mutually exclusive, nor are they intended to describe a serial process with the didactic style being best at the beginning and the heuristic style at the end. As the registrar encounters new experiences, he or she may need to be taught in an earlier style. The key is to be flexible, being sensitive to the needs of the registrar and teaching in a suitable style. Evaluation of your teaching will help indicate if the style was appropriate.

Evaluation

This is about discovering strengths and weaknesses in your teaching so you can decide how well you did and decide where you might want to make changes. Both the trainer and registrar can do this, and it should be an open process. Evaluation produces results that are incorporated into subsequent teaching and is thus an integral part of the tutorial. Just as teaching would not take place without adequate preparation, so there should be no teaching without adequate time being allotted for evaluation.

Six areas can be usefully evaluated:

1 Structure: Was good use made of time? Did both trainer and registrar make adequate preparations?

2 Process: How was the interaction between the registrar and trainer? Was it appropriate? What tended to help the tutorial move on and where and why did it get stuck?

3 Content: Was the content appropriate for the registrar and based on his or her needs rather than the strengths of the trainer? Was it at the right depth for the registrar, and based on previous knowledge and understanding?

4 Style: Was it registrar-led or mainly trainer-centred? What new knowledge, skills and understanding did the registrar develop?

5 Relevance: Was the tutorial relevant to the needs of the registrar, and did it take into account his or her previous knowledge and stage of training?

6 Intentions and achievements: Were the aims and learning outcomes that the trainer and registrar set at the beginning of the tutorial met? Were registrar's needs met? If not, why not, and has time been set aside to address these at a later date?

Many trainers and registrars also note down their feelings about the teaching event. This can help highlight future areas for discussion. The net result of this evaluation is to produce a statement about what action needs to take place in the future, both by the registrar and by the trainer. For example, the trainer may learn that he or she needs to listen more to the needs of the registrar, whereas the registrar may discover that he or she needs to prepare more carefully to maximize the benefits from a tutorial.

The learning cycle

It is clear that evaluation is an essential part of any learning cycle. From evaluation, plans for the next teaching session can be developed. Out of this, aims and objectives for the next tutorial can grow, the trainer and registrar can explore the content of the tutorial, what teaching and learning methods will be used and what resources will be needed.

This spiral process of learning has to take place within the context of the registrar's overall needs as defined in any of the formative assessment programmes, and the organizational needs of the practice and society as a whole. Clear aims for the tutorial can help put these into perspective. Having decided on these broad aims (i.e. what the trainer expects the tutorial to cover), objectives can be agreed. Such objectives can be negotiated between the trainer and registrar at the end of a tutorial. In common with all objectives, they need to be:

- specific
- measurable
- attainable
- realistic
- trackable.

Objectives lead naturally into the style of delivery—bald fact may be best presented didactically, but examination of values is best done in counselling style. Finally, evaluation of the whole tutorial is undertaken, both its process and content, and also a decision is made about what needs to be taught next.

It is also essential to reflect on what the registrar is going to take away from the tutorial that will help him or her subsequently. This is an assessment of change that may result from the tutorial, but is not part of any formal assessment of the registrar as such.

Self-directed learning

Knowles (1990) suggests that adult learning should be based on four assumptions:

1 An adult's self-concept moves from one of being a dependent personality towards being a self-directed human.

2 An adult accumulates an increasing reservoir of experience, which is a rich source of learning.

3 An adult's motivation to learn increases with the relevance of the learning to the developmental tasks or challenges he or she faces.

4 An adult's orientation towards learning shifts from subject-centredness and postponed application of knowledge, to performance-centredness and immediacy of application.

This means that several conditions need to be met in the tutorial if the registrar is to learn most effectively:

1 The registrar should exercise some control and responsibility for the direction of his or her own learning. Ideally the registrar will set the agenda for the tutorial, with the trainer following his or her own agenda when appropriate.

2 The registrar will be able to make use of his or her own experiences as a starting point for the tutorial, and will continue to use these as reference points as the tutorial progresses. It is for this reason that the random-case and problem-case analyses are such effective teaching tools.

3 The registrar needs time, opportunity and guidance to reflect on his or her experiences and turn them into learning experiences.

4 The learning process should be task- or problem-centred. This means that the registrar is dealing with issues that have immediate relevance and application. An example here would be exploring diabetes around diabetic patients whom the registrar has actually seen and the problems encountered, rather than giving a lecture on theoretical aspects of diabetes.

5 Learning should be active. Putting theory into practice early is an ideal way of helping retention and understanding. This means making full use of the learning styles described above.

6 The registrar should be able to share his or her ideas and feelings with the trainer. The registrar should be able to learn from the trainer's experiences and ideas. This means the tutorial must be supportive and the trainer must be able to teach in all teaching styles.

7 The learning climate should be reassuring and conducive to learning. Ideally there should be no anxieties about assessment procedures or fears of criticism from the trainer. This raises real

---

Box 4.2 Conditions for effective learning

- Give registrars some control over their own learning
- Start from their experiences
- Give adequate time for reflection
- Make learning problem-centred
- Make learning active
- Facilitate sharing of experiences
- Enable a supportive environment
- Allow participation in planning tutorials

---

problems for the trainer, who must act as both coach and assessor. There are ways of minimizing these problems. The trainer, for example, can state clearly at the outset when he or she is facilitating and when assessing, reserving assessment for separate sessions. The registrar will, nevertheless, always be aware that the trainer will be looking for areas where improvement could be made. Some trainers ask other trainers to assess the registrar, with the registrar spending time in another practice, where a different trainer assesses their performance.

8 Registrars should be involved in negotiating their own learning. They should be encouraged to accept a share of the responsibility for planning, operating and evaluating the whole tutorial programme for the year. They should also have some choice over the learning methods (Box 4.2).

Learning diaries and logbooks

A written account of the training process is essential for both trainer and registrar. Many regions now supply log diaries in which the registrar can record aspects of his or her training. Formats for this vary from a plain notebook to a very structured format. Some form of written record of training **must** be kept, to record progress and to provide evidence to support the summative assessment process. These records are the property of the registrar, but the trainer must also keep a copy, which, because it is confidential to the registrar and trainer, must be kept secure.

Records of each tutorial will be kept in the logbook. The aims and objectives for each session, intended learning outcomes and evaluation will also be recorded. There will also be space for the registrar to record details of surgery consultations that he or she would like to learn more about. Many logbooks also have pages to record details of audits carried out, an outline of the registrar's project, summaries of key reading material and difficult cases they have come across.

A learning diary has a different purpose from that of a logbook. It is intended as a journal to help reflective practice, helping individual professional development. There are no special rules for keeping a learning diary. It is a personal document that is intended to be read by and reflected on by the registrar only. The registrar is asked to reflect on each day, noting meaningful recollections. Whereas the logbook is intended to record more factual information, the diary is less structured and is used to capture impressions and feelings.

The diary is not to be offered for judgement or interpretation by others, and it certainly forms no part in assessment or evaluation. It reflects on the developing process of being a registrar. It records the development of an individual as a professional, helping them to examine both the joys and the difficulties. This process helps in reflection, an integral part of being a sound practitioner.

Keeping a diary involves a cyclical pattern of reflection, first reflecting on experiences in the process of writing and then reflecting back on the diary entries themselves. Revisiting the experiences and the emotions these brought up at the time can be painful, but it allows attitudes and beliefs about particular experiences to be re-examined. Reflection will force us to examine behaviour, which may then involve acceptance, analysis and change. Reflection on experiences, and our perceptions of them at the time, forces us to review our behaviour, without moulding it into good or bad, right or wrong. It also forces us to reflect on what is and what is not important, and helps to get balance into a rushed, pressured professional life.

Conclusion

The tutorial should be one of the most enjoyable and rewarding parts of working with a registrar. It is a time for sharing knowledge and skills, for sharing experiences, the joys and the sadnesses of working as a GP. It moves beyond apprenticeship into the world of adult learning, developing with the registrar methods of learning that will stand him or her in good stead for ever. To offer a good tutorial is challenging, requires work, preparation and evaluation. But doing it well offers the registrar an incomparably rich learning experience.

References

Honey, P. & Mumford, A. (1986) *The Manual of Learning Style.*

Knowles, M. (1990) *The Adult Learner: a Neglected Species*, 4th edn. Gulf Publishing, Houston.

Kolb, D. & Fry, R. (1975) Towards an applied theory of experiential learning. In: *Theories of Group Processes* (ed. C. Cooper). John Wiley, Chichester.

Luft, J. & Harrington, I. (1984) *Group Process: An Introduction to Group Dynamics.* Mayfield Publishers, Palo Alto, CA.

Morton, L.T. & Wright, D.J. (1990) *How to Use a Medical Library*, 7th edn. Library Association Publishing Ltd, London.

Royal College of General Practitioners (1972) *The Future General Practitioner—Learning and Teaching.* RCGP, London.

5 Consultation skills

Introduction

To be able to talk to, understand and explain to our patients are basic skills. To be an effective GP we have to see these abilities as important and be prepared to work at them. However, it is not just the skills that are important, our attitudes to our patients and our goals are of equal importance. Consultation skills are a means to an end, we have to decide what outcomes we wish to achieve. The logical sequence must be: what tasks need to be completed, what strategies could be used and, then, what skills will be needed to complete the task.

Our attitudes are important, because our behaviours tend to follow. If we believe in involving patients in decision making, as is fashionable, we will use consulting strategies and skills to that end. If the opposite view is held, prevalent for most of medicine's recorded history, that withholding knowledge, maintaining mystique and instructing patients without involving them is the most effective way of practising, then we are hardly likely to value, learn or practise strategies and skills for involving them in decision making. What attitudes or opinions do you have about communicating with your patients? Do you favour involvement? Is it better to share or to tell? Think about it.

What do we need to achieve in our consultations?

The following list of tasks is taken from the MRCGP statement of clinical and consulting competence:
- Discover the reasons for a patient's attendance.
- Define the clinical problem(s).
- Address the patient's problem(s).
- Explain the problem(s) to the patient.
- Make effective use of the consultation.

These five consulting requirements are too broad to be of real help within the consulting room and need elaborating. As an example, the further tasks that need to be completed, in order to obtain a clear picture of why our patient has come to us are listed below:

- Elicit the patient's account of the symptom(s) that made him or her turn to us.
- Obtain relevant items of social and occupational circumstances.
- Determine the patient's health understanding.
- Enquire about other continuing problems.

Strategies and skills—how best can we elicit our patient's account?

The patient's account can be elicited most effectively by:
- Encouraging the patient's contribution throughout the consultation.
- Picking up, as far as our skills allow, the many communication cues that the patient gives us.

As you see these requirements are skilful but they have not prescribed the skills you might use.

The simplest way to do this is to let the patient talk, actively encourage his or her contribution to the consultation, watch your patient all the time they are talking. Look for cues, verbal and non-verbal, try not to interrupt too much. Use your perceptive faculties to actually hear what they are saying and try to pick up the message behind the message.

There are good reasons for letting the patient have a minute or two of relatively uninterrupted dialogue at the beginning of a consultation. The first is that, contrary to what you may think, it often **saves time**. The reasons why letting the patient talk can save time are related, first, to the patient's agenda and, second, to yours.

The patient, and **only** the patient, knows why he or she has come to you. If you start on your agenda too soon, you may never discover the fear of cancer, the fear of the effects of expected therapy, but, more importantly, you may not discover what it is that the patient wants to know.

Establishing your patient's agenda early on allows you to

negotiate the use of time in the consultation, to agree on what will be dealt with now and what can be left for another day.

Picking up on the cues that our patients give us is a skill all doctors need to develop—these are the signposts to the hidden, or not so hidden, agendas. No GP can hope to be effective or get job satisfaction without developing an ability to use cues and having a feeling of when to act and when to wait.

In 1994 the *American Journal of Pediatrics* published a paper that contained the Holy Grail of communication skills. The three skills that improved patient's disclosure of sensitive information were found to be:

1 Asking questions about psychological issues. For example: 'What frightened you?', 'Did that make you feel depressed?'

2 Making supportive statements. For example: 'That must have been hard but you seem to have managed very well.'

3 Listening attentively.

The expression **active listening** is now often used; a number of suggestions for things to try are listed below:

- Let the patient talk first and set the agenda. **Beginnings are very important** and will affect the course of the whole meeting. Start in an open manner, not closed. Think of the difference between 'Hello, well now?' with a smile and a raised eyebrow, as opposed to 'It's your blood pressure, isn't it, up with the sleeve.' Even the standard opening of 'Hello, what can I do for you' is controlling, implying an action. You may think this is nit-picking, but do experiment with the effects of various opening gambits. Like playing a game of chess, you can win or lose the consultation in the first few exchanges.
- Show that you are listening, focus on your patient, make eye contact. Comments can help, such as: 'You look sad today'; 'That must have been very frightening'; 'How did that make you feel?', etc.
- Actively encourage your patient to talk. Nod, smile and echo significant words.
- Repeat tentatively, in your own words, your understanding of the patient's story.
- Reflect back, not only to show that you understand, but also to enable the patient to hear and understand his or her own meaning.
- Try again if you do not seem to be getting anywhere.

- Allow silences, the patient will almost invariably fill them.
- Watch for verbal and non-verbal clues.
- Use open questions. These are good for beliefs, they cannot be answered yes or no. For example: 'Tell me about...'; 'What is it like?...'; 'What are you worried about?'..., etc. If you are having difficulty getting the patient to tell you what really matters, the easiest way to obtain better results is to regularly use the phrase 'Tell me more'—patients usually will.
- Explain why you are asking a question, this can stimulate revealing responses: 'The reason I asked about wind and bloating was I was wondering about irritable bowel syndrome'; 'Oh my sister's got that and she said that's what I've got but my mother reckons it's an ulcer.'

Here are some common failings to try to avoid:

- Talking too much about youself.
- Making too many well-intentioned comments too early on.
- Echoing the patient's last words can be helpful but too much parroting is not.
- Do not pretend to have understood if you have not.
- Resist filling in the silences yourself.

You must search for the patient's beliefs—his or her ideas, concerns, expectations, feelings and the effects. Attempt to allow the patient to voice his or her real concern. This means more than just active listening; it means being interested, wanting to know. To be a good doctor you have to care about people; if your patient understands that, he or she will in turn tell you what they care about. Ask the same sort of questions the patient has asked him- or herself. Why has this patient come? Why now? What has happened? Why has it happened? Why to him or her? Try to put yourself in the patient's shoes.

What about the frequently discussed **empathy**? Empathy is a much-abused concept. The idea behind empathy is to identify mentally with the patient, and so fully comprehend him or her. This is fine as long as you realize it is only an aim that can help you communicate with the patient. To succeed in fully empathizing with anybody is impossible. How can middle class GPs really empathize with drug-abusing teenagers. We can be compassionate and we can care for them but the vast majority of us will be unable to empathize with them.

Here are a few more eliciting skills to think about:
- Speak the patient's language, do not talk down, and avoid jargon. This implies we have a feel for the patient's language in the first place—you have to work at that. Patronizing 'doctor speak' should be a form of communication that dies with this century, but that may be wishful thinking. Jargon is ingrained in doctors to such an extent that we often do not realize what is seen to be jargon to our patients. Keep looking at your own performance and pick out the words and sentences that need translating.
- Remember that closed questions are good for pigeon-holing facts and pattern recognition and bad for beliefs and feelings. Closed questions tend to increase doctor control, and they can only be answered very specifically, often with just a yes or a no. For example: 'Is it painful?'; 'Are your bowels OK?'

Involving patients

The patient should be involved in choosing his or her own management as much as possible, not least because it will depend on the patient for the plan to be implemented. Management options should be shared with the patient and, where appropriate, he or she should make the choice.

You may initially find this concept uncomfortable, but it is likely to make you more effective and less prone to create disease out of what may essentially be a problem of living. Encourage the patient to be responsible for his or her own health. This may enable the patient to be more in control of his or her own health destiny and thus more likely to request information, as well as to use the medical profession more appropriately. If the patient is involved, the risk of litigation and disagreement is much less.

How to improve your negotiating skills

A number of steps can be taken to improve your negotiating skills:
- You make the first move. You have to outline your position and your reasons.
- Think aloud and state your position, be honest. Perhaps 'fly some kites' to give the patient a choice.

- Ask the patient what he or she thinks. Find out his or her position. To help with this watch the 'internal search', if you do not see the patient looking like they will accept, keep negotiating. Watch for 'non-verbal leakage'. This sounds like a pool of muddy water forming around the patient, but it actually means a discrepancy between what the patient says and what his or her non-verbal behaviour is indicating. For example: 'No I'm not depressed Doc', while sitting, shoulders slumped, with a sad fixed expression and exuding gloom; or 'Yes I will try the tablets, probably', while shiftily breaking eye contact and squirming in the chair. You have to act on these cues to be effective. For example: 'I know you say you are not depressed but you do look it to me, are you sure there isn't something I can help with?'.

When involving the patient in decision making, remember to:
- Counter the patient's fallacious arguments and erroneous beliefs.
- Reinforce those beliefs that are helpful to the outcome.

Some strategies for getting patients to do what is good for them (for example, giving up smoking, losing weight, taking tablets)

Make things easy. People are more likely to do things if there are fewer things to do, if they fit existing patterns of living and if they have the resources to do them.

Think of the context. People are likely to do things if they do them with other people, if they are reminded at the time to do them, if they know someone might be likely to check to see if they have been done and if the people they live and work with help them.

Think of the patient's perceptions. People are more likely to do things that seem important, and when they understand why they should do them and how to do them. If they really believe, they will follow your advice, but they are more likely to do things if their anxiety level is moderate and not high.

Think of the relationship. People are more likely to do things if they have helped to decide to do them. If they have promised to do them, if they have faith in you their doctor, especially if they think you like and respect them, and they are more likely to do things they are rewarded for doing.

Explaining

Share your findings with the patient

Always try to explain your working diagnosis, what management options seem appropriate and what the possible effects of any treatment are likely to be.

Tailor the explanation to the needs of the patient

By now you have got to know the patient a little. You should have a feel for the sort of person he or she is, so when you begin to explain ensure that your manner and language seem appropriate to what the patient needs and is likely to understand. Your explanation should be linked to the patient's beliefs that you elicited earlier. This does not mean you have to adopt all of the patient's beliefs; some may be quite erroneous. However, you must make your explanation bespoke, not off the peg—individually tailored to that unique human sitting in front of you. This will make it enormously more relevant than the standard hysterectomy spiel or the routine explanation about irritable bowels.

Ensure that explanations are understood and accepted by the patient

Doctors, on balance, are quite good at giving explanations. The fly in the ointment is that patients are bad at understanding them. Watch your peers explaining to patients and ask yourself, are they explaining for their patient's benefit or their own? Many explanations seem more for the doctor's benefit than for the patient's. Ask yourself, am I explaining for me or for my patient?

What you are trying to achieve is a **shared understanding** and this is different from a simple explanation. The danger is of making the explanation a one-way process: 'I am the full vessel and I will pour my knowledge into the empty vessel that is my patient.' This does not work; it has to be a two-way process.

Strategies for explaining and achieving shared understanding

A number of strategies for explaining and achieving shared understanding are listed below:

- Elicit the patient's beliefs; you cannot share unless you have something to share.
- It is necessary to translate and share your medical knowledge honestly and with respect for the patient.
- Be prepared to admit uncertainty. This can be difficult, for both doctor and patient.
- Clarify how much information the patient would like to know about his or her condition. This is a skilful strategy and needs practising.
- Do not reassure too soon. This can be interpreted as rejection, or just as valueless if the patient is convinced that you do not have the information needed.
- At all times remember that an explanation is a one-way process. Sharing understanding is the goal you are aiming for and is a two-way behaviour.

Explaining skills

A number of these skills are detailed below:

- Information should be presented without the use of jargon, using short words and sentences as specifically as possible.
- The order of presentation counts. Patients recall best what they are told first.
- Important items should be repeated.
- Provide explicit categorization. For example, 'I am going to tell you what I think is wrong, what I expect to happen, and what treatment I suggest.' This is a bit military but very effective.
- Use leaflets, tapes, laser disks, Health line, etc. Do read or listen to them first, you may find you disagree vehemently; ideally write them yourself.
- Encourage feedback and keep checking the patient's understanding.
- Do not give too much information. This means not getting carried away with your own verbosity. A patient staring out of the windows at the squirrels is a sure sign that you have gone on for too long.

- Climb down a few steps from your pedestal. In other words try not to be too distanced from the patient because of your need to be professional.
- Use similar phrases to those of the patient and some of his or her own descriptions.
- Share a little of yourself from time to time. For example: 'I had an operation once'; 'Migraines are bloody awful, aren't they?'
- Show understanding and empathy.
- Be prepared to back down. Achieving a shared understanding does not mean getting the patient to always agree with you. It means that to achieve a genuine sharing you may have to agree with the patient. This may make you uneasy.
- Keep a dialogue going—you cannot share with a monologue.

How to make effective use of the consultation

Use of time

Perhaps the most precious resource of all is time. Make efficient and sensible use of available time and, if necessary, recommend further consultations as appropriate. The use of time by doctors is a subtle area of study. It is not the length of time that is so important but the use to which the time is put. In general practice it probably takes a minimum of eight well-used minutes to achieve a reasonable degree of shared management and shared understanding. There have been many studies carried out on time with patients in all sorts of settings; interestingly, it emerges that the amount of time spent does not seem to significantly affect patient satisfaction. This should remind us that it is the use to which we put the time that matters. Some doctors can waffle away for 15 minutes with no difficulty, while others can be patient-focused and enquire efficiently within half that timescale.

Establishing an effective relationship with the patient

The word effective is the crux here, what you wish to achieve is a relationship that helps you to complete the other tasks. You must discover the reasons for the patient's attendance, define the clinical problem, address the patient's problem, explain effectively and make overall effective use of the consultation. How you achieve this is your business. You may well have been taught interpersonal skills, such as empathizing, eye contact, use of touch and so on. These skills are very useful but must not be used without thinking of what you wish to achieve. We have all met lovely, warm, empathetic doctors who are frankly ineffective, and we have also come across some pretty unpleasant cold fish who are effective.

There are of course some styles of behaviour that are more likely to produce an effective relationship than others, not least a genuine show of interest in the patient as a fellow human, but there is no one style that will suit all. Concentrate on your strengths and what you feel comfortable with and work on your effectiveness.

Opportunistic health-promotion advice

The point at issue here is do you take an appropriate moment in the consultation to give such advice?

Linking lifestyle advice to a current illness can be quite an effective way of altering behaviour. Just telling patients to stop smoking and giving them a leaflet will mean between 5% and 10% will give up, an astonishingly high figure if you think of how many patients you see. The consultation does provide the opportunity for such advice, but, **most importantly**, not to the exclusion of the patient's agenda.

Strategies for making effective use of the consultation

The following strategies will help to make effective use of the consultation:

- Determine the reasons for the patient's attendance at the outset. This then allows you both to set the agenda, what you will cover today and what can be reasonably left for another occasion. This is a genuinely time-conserving strategy.
- Determine the patient's own ideas, concerns and expectations before attempting an explanation, so lessening the risk of a 'dysfunctional' consultation. This also means the explanation becomes tailored to that individual patient.
- Use each consultation as part of a learning circle; thus some tasks can be achieved over a series of consultations. The adop-

tion of these methods may also change the patient's expectations about the appropriate use of time and resources.
- Help the patient to appreciate the costs and benefits of compliance and non-compliance.
- Share most management options.

Skills helpful for making effective use of the consultation

The use of the following skills will make the consultation more effective:
- General communication skills. Several recent studies have shown that a female style of communication in consultations results in more sharing and better outcomes. This applies with patients of both sexes. What this means for male doctors, myself included, is food for thought, but men may have to acknowledge that the more participative female style has a certain merit that lessons can be learned from.
- Skills of appropriate control (for example: judicious use of doctor authority to control speech flow; appropriate use of negative non-verbal behaviour, such as **not** looking at the patient) will tend to staunch the flow. Closing the notes can signal the end of the consultation.
- Be friendly and attentive, adopt an informal style. However, be wary of the overuse of first names, it is easy to be patronizing. After a while it is not unreasonable to ask your patient if he or she minds the use of first names. Many patients quite like being called by their first name but they will never call you by yours. Be careful when using the notes in this type of situation, as use of the first name indicated may be fraught with dangers—a Mr Cyril Jones may hate being called Cyril and with his friends will only answer to Jack; you, however, by not checking have been blithely annoying him for a decade.
- Learn to recognize the effect of your own behaviour on the patient. Are you frightening? Do you inspire trust? Do your patients come back to you? What do they tell you about yourself?
- Learn to recognize, interpret and use your feelings. You are feeling uneasy and anxious: is the patient feeling that way to? You are getting angry: is the patient angry as well?
- Learn to recognize and deal with your own stress.

	What was done well and why?	How could it be done better?
Discover the reasons for a patient's attendance Elicit the patient's account of the symptoms Encourage the patient's contribution Observe and use cues Obtain relevant items of social and occupational circumstances Explore the patient's health understanding		
Define the clinical problems		
Explain the problems to the patient Explain the diagnosis management and effects of treatment Use appropriate language Use the patient's health understanding Check understanding		
Manage the patient's problem Make sure the plan is appropriate for the working diagnosis Share the management options		
Effectiveness Use time appropriately Prescribe appropriately Develop and use your relationship Opportunistic health advice		

Figure 5.1 A consultation critique sheet.

An example of a form that you can use to review your consultations is given in Fig. 5.1. You will find it more useful to fill in those areas in which you felt you did well first, and then the areas you felt you could have done better in. If there is a lot in the first column and nothing too drastic in the second, then that looks like a consultation worth including in any assessment.

Further reading

Balint, M. (1957) *The Doctor, His Patient and the Illness.* Tavistock Publications, London.

Becker, M. *et al.* (1979) Patient perceptions and compliance: recent studies of the health belief model. In: *Compliance in Health Care.* Johns Hopkins University Press, Baltimore.

Benson, J. & Britten, N. (1996) Respecting the autonomy of cancer patients when talking with their families. *British Medical Journal* **313**, 729–731.

Byrne, P. & Long, B. (1976) *Doctors Talking to Patients.* HMSO, London.

Cromarty, I. (1996) What do patients think about during their consultations? An interesting qualitative study demonstrating that patients routinely consider their relationship with us doctors, and assess if we are in a good mood, are not too tired, etc., and alter their behaviour accordingly. *British Journal of General Practice* **46**, 525–528.

Fitzpatrick, R. (1996) Telling patients there is nothing wrong. *British Medical Journal* **313**, 311.

Ford, S., Fallowfield, L. & Lewis, S. (1996) Doctor–patient interactions in oncology. *Social Science and Medicine* **42**, 1511–1519.

Greenfield, S., Kaplan, S.H., Ware, J.E., Jr, Yano, E.M. & Frank, H.J. (1988) Patient's participation in medical care: effects of blood sugar and control and quality of life in diabetes. *Journal of General Internal Medicine* **88**, 448–457.

Kai, J. (1996a) Parents' difficulties and information needs in coping with acute illness in pre-school children: a qualitative study. *British Medical Journal* **313**, 987–990.

Kai, J. (1996b) What worries parents when their pre-school children are acutely ill, and why: a qualitative study. *British Medical Journal* **313**, 983–986.

Ley, P. (1988) *Communicating with Patients.* Croom Helm, London.

Little, P., Williamson, I., Warner, G., Gould, C., Gantley, M. & Kinmonth, A.-L. (1997) Open randomised trial of prescribing strategies in managing sore throat. *British Medical Journal* **314**, 722–727.

McDonald, I.G., Daly, J., Jelinek, V.M., Panetta, F. & Gutman, J.M. (1996) Opening Pandora's box: the unpredictability of reassurance by a normal test result. *British Medical Journal* **313**, 329–332.

Makoul, G., Arnston, P. & Schofield, T. (1995) Health promotion in primary care: physician–patient communication and decision making about prescription medications. *Social Science and Medicine* **41**, 1241–1254.

Martin, E., Russell, D., Goodwin, S., Chapman, R., North, M. & Sheridan, P. (1991) Why patient's consult and what happens when they do. *British Medical Journal* **303**, 289–292.

Meredith, C., Symonds, P., Webster, L. *et al.* (1996) Information needs of cancer patients in west Scotland: cross sectional survey of patients' views. *British Medical Journal* **313**, 724–726.

Neighbour, R. (1987) *The Inner Consultation. How to Develop an Effective and Intuitive Consulting Style.* Librapharm Ltd, Newbury, UK.

Pendleton, D., Schofield, T., Tate, P. & Havelock, P. (1984) *The Consultation. An Approach to Learning and Teaching.* Oxford University Press, Oxford.

Savage, R. & Armstrong, D. (1990) Effect of a GP's consulting style on patient's satisfaction: controlled study. *British Medical Journal* **301**, 968–970.

Silverman, J., Kurtz, S. & Draper, J. (1998) *Skills for Communicating with Patients.* Radcliffe Medical Press, Abingdon, UK.

Stott, N. & Davis, R.H. (1979) The exceptional potential in each primary care consultation. *Journal of the Royal College of General Practitioners* **29**, 201–205.

Tate, P. (1997) *The Doctor's Communication Handbook*, 2nd edn. Radcliffe Press, Oxford.

Tuckett, D., Boulton, M., Olson, C. & Williams, A. (1985) *Meetings Between Experts.* Tavistock Publications, London.

Waitzkin, H. & Stoeckle, J.D. (1972) The communication of information about illness. *Advances in Psychosomatic Medicine* **8**, 180–215.

Wilson, A. (1991) Consultation length in general practice: a review. *British Journal of General Practice* **41**, 119–122.

6 The vocational training scheme course

What is the vocational training scheme (VTS) all about? Is what happens on the half-day-release course a secret? What **does** happen on the half-day-release course? What are course organizers and what do they do? How can I find out more? Am I allowed to know more?

These questions, and many more like them, will have occurred to trainers and GP registrars who want to know more about training for general practice, and in particular more about their local VTS and what it can do. After the introduction of compulsory vocational training 16 years ago, many trainers will have experienced a VTS at first hand, but change affects all areas and this includes vocational training and the methods and skills used on the courses. Established trainers may therefore not be entirely sure about how their local VTS is working. Potential GP registrars will only know what they hear from the senior house officers (SHOs) working with them during their preregistration year, unless they make an effort to discover more. Even current GP registrars may not be aware of everything that is happening on their course, so this source of information may not be entirely valid for making a decision about a particular VTS.

Communication is therefore an important responsibility for all those involved in a VTS, and course organizers have a special role in maintaining good relationships with their general practice and hospital colleagues at all levels.

Background

Vocational training started in the early 1970s, but was not compulsory until 1981 and was not compulsory for the full 3 years until 1982. Two years in recognized hospital posts and 1 year in a training practice are the current requirements, although in some parts of the country it is possible to spend 18 months of the 3 years in general practice.

During the 3-year programme, GP registrars have the opportunity to attend the half-day-release course run in their area. These VTSs are recognized as an important part of training for general practice and are monitored by a national system of supervision, which is the responsibility of the Joint Committee on Postgraduate Training for General Practice (JCPTGP). These courses are run by appointed course organizers, who are responsible to the regional adviser in general practice, now known as the educational director.

The structure of the scheme

Schemes vary in their approach, from arranging a full 3-year programme to organizing practice attachments and a training programme for 1 year only. Many schemes are flexible enough to be able to arrange most combinations of training that may be needed.

Some schemes arrange a half-day-release educational programme throughout the whole of the 3 years and others will arrange a programme only during the GP training year. There are arguments for and against each approach. A 3-year programme allows much more ground to be covered, and allows GP registrars to be introduced to the theories of adult education in a pragmatic way over a reasonable period. Drawbacks include the problems of getting away from the wards to attend, and the subsequent problems with disrupted small groups if attendance is infrequent. Such disadvantages are not normally a problem during the practice attachment, but if this is the only time during the 3 years for a half-day-release programme then the advantages of using adult-educational and small-group theory are reduced.

Other disadvantages of a 1-year course include the loss of continuous contact with other GP registrars and course organizers, and the lack of information in the hospital years about courses and examinations best undertaken in that time.

Most VTSs are run in the local postgraduate medical centre, where there is usually an experienced secretary, who is available to answer questions about the scheme and advise potential and existing GP registrars whenever possible. It is much easier to contact the secretary than the course organizers, who are active GPs working part time in postgraduate education, but the secretary will refer problems and queries to course organizers if he or she is not personally able to help.

The course organizer's role

Course organizers are appointed after interview and have usually been trainers before their appointment. This means that they all have experience of educational techniques and most have experience of working in small groups, which is the commonest format for a half-day-release scheme.

A brief outline of the job description for a course organizer includes a wide range of requirements and skills. Educational expertise is needed for curriculum planning, assessment, facilitating small groups, guidance on topic presentations and encouraging GP registrars to take responsibility for their own programme. Communication skills are needed for liaising with GP trainers, hospital consultants, hospital administrators and the GP registrars themselves, not to mention the various secretaries and visitors involved. Other roles include organizing interviews for appointments to the VTS, arranging hospital and training practice attachments and organizing the necessary courses that GP registrars expect, such as MRCGP, family planning and practice management courses.

A VTS is not static and the continuing development of the scheme is an important part of a course organizer's work.

Communication with trainers

Activities on the half-day release are certainly not secret and trainers really need to know what is being taught so that they can plan their own teaching programme with their registrars. There is no ruling which says that GP registrars cannot discuss their half-day release with their trainer, but it is surprising how often trainers say that they have no clear idea about what is being taught. It is a responsibility of course organizers to inform trainers about their course content, but trainers can be active in this and ask their GP registrar or approach a course organizer directly. Most course organizers have links with the local trainers' workshop, and this is an excellent place to exchange information. Copies of termly programmes can also be sent to every trainer via their GP registrar, so there is no excuse for trainers not being informed about the programme.

What should be taught where?

In training practices the relationship is usually one to one, so that a teaching programme specific for an individual GP registrar can be made. The programme will depend on the GP registrar's identified learning needs; although there will be some areas of ignorance common to all GP registrars, there will be many more areas where knowledge and skills will vary widely from one person to another. The VTS cannot realistically identify each GP registrar's training needs and tailor a programme to match. However, it **can** devise a programme to meet GP registrar needs, such as communication skills and attitude issues, which are best met using small peer-group teaching methods.

Facts can be learned from books and formal lectures, but the application of those facts in a working situation is often better learned in a small-group environment, where there is more than one person with whom to discuss problems. Very often the same topic can be discussed with a trainer as well as on the VTS, but the perspective will be different. The GP registrar will learn more about how his or her views compare with the peers on the VTS and will learn more about the practical issues in discussion with the trainer. Random and problem case analyses (see below) will also have a different emphasis in each setting.

Thus the trainer will tailor a programme that is much more specific to GP registrars than the VTS can provide, and the VTS can respond to the needs of a whole group.

The relevance of adult educational theory

In modern education adults and children usually learn in different ways—children learn and are taught in a teacher-centred way, known as pedagogy, and adult learning takes into account pre-vious experience and knowledge, which children do not have. Adult learning is therefore learner-centred and is known as andro-gogy. It is as important for trainers as it is for course organizers to be aware of the implications of basic adult educational theory, so that when GP registrars question the methods used on the half-day-release scheme they understand and can explain what is happening.

Knowles (1970) has proposed this model of the adult learner:
- He or she is self-directed but has a conditioned expectation to be dependent and to be taught.
- He or she has previous experience so that quite often the most appropriate resource for adult learning is a group of similar adult learners.
- Adults learn better when there is a good reason for learning.
- Most adults do not learn for the sake of learning, but because they have a problem to solve or a task to complete.

This implies that adult learning involves applying experiential learning to similar life situations, rather than learning units of fact. The relevance of the learning is therefore more easily identified by the learners and stimulates their own involvement in learning by encouraging them to:
- be involved in curriculum planning with their teachers
- identify their own learning needs
- define their own aims
- plan their own learning
- assess their own learning.

Rogers (1988) summarized the principles of adult learning in his comment: 'The purpose of adult education is to help them to learn, not to teach them all they know and thus stop them from carrying on learning.' There is a difference, therefore, between abrogation of the teacher's responsibility and delegation to the learners. It is the teacher's role to delegate increasing responsibil-ity to his or her adult pupils while recognizing that the learners will still need his or her help.

Gray (1977), in his 'educational triangle' (Fig. 6.1), outlined the principles of planning individual educational sessions or courses.

This educational triangle provides a way of answering the questions:

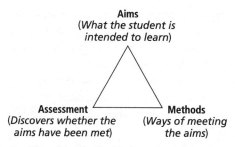

Figure 6.1 The educational triangle.

1 What do I want the students to learn by the end of the session (or course)?

2 How can I teach them what I want them to learn?

3 Have they learned what I intended?

Using a model like this can help course organizers and trainers to plan their teaching more effectively.

All these principles apply to teaching in the practice as well as on the half-day-release scheme.

Working in a group

Using small peer groups in education is not a new idea in medical education and the Royal College of General Practitioners (1972) has advocated small-group work in training GPs for over 30 years.

Learning groups have the defined aim of being educational for each member and helping with the development of appropriate knowledge, skills and attitudes, according to the specific objectives of the group. A significant amount of learning will occur through discussion between members of the group, and for this reason learning groups are frequently called discussion groups. The terms are interchangeable. It is usual to define an educational group as a collection of people with the main aim of learning in each of the three main fields (knowledge, skills and attitude). The group will need to know why it is meeting to be properly effective. Johnson and Johnson (1991) identified the following important points that are necessary for a discussion group to work well:

- Clear goals.
- Good mutual communication.

- Widespread participation and leadership among members.
- Use of consensus to reach answers, solutions and decisions.
- Power and influence based on expertise and access to information and skills, not authority.
- The frequent occurrence of controversy.
- Open confrontation, and negotiation of conflicts of interest, among members and between members and the group facilitator.
- High cohesiveness (group identity).
- High trust among members.
- A supportive climate among members and facilitator.
- Group 'norms' encouraging individual responsibility and accountability, helping and sharing, and achievement.
- Good group and interpersonal skills among members.

Group members need to realize that all these points are important and should be encouraged to learn the basic skills and attitudes that will help their group to become more productive and achieve its full potential.

Group development

Most discussion groups progress through a number of stages during their development before reaching a really effective stage. Tuckman (1965) described the stages of group development after reviewing a large number of studies on group development:

1 Forming stage: in which members are uncertain about the structure and function of the group and try to determine rules and procedures while defining their own placing in the group.

2 Storming stage: in which conflicts arise as members of the group rebel against the group task and try to establish their own independence.

3 Norming stage: in which the group decides on its own rules for behaviour, and cohesiveness and commitment to the group are founded.

4 Performing stage: in which goals are achieved and the group develops flexible and positive ways of working together.

As stage 4 is reached, group members begin to realize that it is their own aims that are being met by the group process. The success of the group work is therefore their own success, built on the first three stages of their development. In the early stages it is the group facilitator (course organizer) who guides the group, helping with the setting of goals and establishment of procedures. The storming phase is necessary for group members to learn that they have the ability to direct their own learning and to take responsibility for that. Therefore in the last two stages the group has taken over responsibility for its function and recognized that the aims and objectives are theirs. In this way the 'ownership' of the group gradually changes from the facilitator to the group itself.

GP registrars often have difficulty working in groups under these circumstances, because they have not experienced such a style of education before. It is right that they should question the methodology and also right that those involved in the teaching are aware of the theory that supports the practice. The most difficult time for all concerned can be during the storming phase, when emotions can affect the content of the programme. At this time a most effective way of helping the GP registrars is to allow them time to express their feelings and explain the reasons for adopting a small-group approach.

The emphasis eventually becomes learner-centred or focused, so that the groups, and the individuals in the group, have their own learning needs met. The implication for course organizers and trainers is that flexibility is essential. What one group or GP registrar needs may not be right for another.

What is it like to be in a VTS group?

This depends on the approach adopted by the course organizers for the scheme and on the previous experience of individual GP registrars. Undergraduate medical education is changing, especially within departments of general practice, and it is there that students are most likely to have experienced the kind of teaching and group work that is frequently used on a VTS half-day-release course.

Course organizers will have decided on the teaching methods they will use for the course they have planned and they will have developed their own small-group leadership skills to a varying degree. The course organizer who knows everything about general practice has never existed but he or she will know about educational methods and how to use them. Small peer groups in this context are not actually led but are facilitated. The difference is significant and reflects the role of the group facilitator as someone who guides the group but does not give the answers sought.

Small-group work can seem frustrating at first, almost as if the group is left to sort itself out with very little help from the course organizer. Anyone not used to the approach will quickly encourage a move into the storming phase described above. This can be threatening and emotions are evident, which can discourage some group members. A skilled facilitator will know how to help the group through the storming phase with a positive outcome. There is no easy way to move through this most difficult of the phases, but the group members learn that conflict can be positive and that avoiding conflict is a barrier to understanding what is happening in a relationship and to trying to understand other people and oneself.

Once the storming phase is over, groups will become more productive and group members will become more relaxed and learn in an atmosphere that is safe but not necessarily without disagreement or argument.

A GP registrar who has previous experience of group work may be aware of what is happening, but most are not. Understanding what is going on, and why it is going on, helps tremendously. This knowledge is used to help increase communication skills, which in turn can make the consultation more productive. The message is that group work can be stimulating and rewarding but at times it can feel uncomfortable and threatening. Good group facilitators are able to make the discomfort productive and they will normally be able to help the group help themselves. Self-directed learning with learner-focused teaching is the result.

Teaching methods used

Small-group work is the norm for most schemes but a lecture format is the most efficient way of disseminating facts and lectures or 'lecturettes' may be used as well. Most teaching methods centre on the small groups and will include group discussion, role-play, random- and problem-case analysis, presentations by group members and video analysis.

Group discussion

The backbone of group work is the discussion within the group. This may be based on a specific topic agreed or identified by group members, or based on something that has happened in the group. There is no limit to the possibilities, and the group facilitator will ensure the process is educational and relevant. Topics that may be discussed can be factual or behavioural (task-related or process-related).

Lecturettes, short presentations by a group member, can also form the basis of group discussion.

Role-play

A simple way of finding out what it is like to be a patient, and therefore understanding patients' fears and problems, is to become involved in role-play. The group facilitator or a group member will devise situations based on real life, which one group member role-playing the general practitioner will try to resolve. Another group member will role-play the patient, with others playing family members as necessary. The rest of the group observes the whole process and then discusses the consultation, using Pendleton's Rules (Pendleton, 1984), which are outlined in Box 6.1. This is a

---

Box 6.1 A précis of Pendleton's Rules

1 The presenting doctor explains the situation of the consultation.
2 The consultation is watched in silence.
3 The presenting doctor answers any questions about matters of fact.
4 The presenting doctor then identifies what he thought he did well in the consultation.
5 The group members (or tutor) identify what they saw being done well.
6 The presenting doctor next identifies what he thought he could have improved on in the consultation.
7 The group members (or tutor) identify what they thought could have been improved on in the consultation.
8 The presenting doctor is given necessary support from the group or tutor.

very useful teaching method, as it is possible to look at how the doctor and patient actually felt during the consultation. Most role-players are surprised at how real they found the situation they were in to be, and the discussion is therefore able to elucidate real patient and doctor feelings in the safe environment of the group.

Case analysis

This is useful for increasing consultation skills and self-awareness.

There are two kinds of case analysis frequently used, and two methods of presenting the cases. Random-case analysis involves choosing at random a case from a surgery brought by a group member. The ensuing discussion can include any aspect of the consultation and practice organization.

Problem-case analysis involves the presenter choosing a case he or she has found difficult. Discussion can be wide but is concentrated on analysing the problem identified. It is not unusual for the actual problem to be quite different from the presented one by the time discussion has finished.

Cases can be presented using the actual notes from a surgery, or by using a video recording of the surgery. The use of video and consultation skills are described in Chapters 3 and 5 respectively.

Other methods used

Depending on the aim for a session, groups can be split into quartets, trios or pairs for a task to be carried out and presented to the whole group. These are sometimes referred to as 'buzz groups'.

Brainstorming is a technique in which group members call out ideas related to the issue under discussion, with the important rule that no idea is discussed or commented on until the brainstorm has finished. Only then is the value of the items on the brainstorm list discussed.

Occasionally the group discussion will be recorded on video, for the group to analyse later in the afternoon. There are several different ways of doing this, one of the most popular and enjoyable is to base the group discussion on an exercise that is not necessarily medical, such as surviving a plane crash in the desert.

The aim is to demonstrate to group members the behaviour occurring in the group, both their own and others'.

The curriculum

Educational theory outlines the necessity of having aims and objectives. A curriculum is important in providing a method of achieving the aims. In an examination-based system (summative assessment), the curriculum will be almost the same as the syllabus that defines precisely the topics to be covered so that students have the greatest chance of passing the exam. In a formative assessment system the curriculum will be a guide to the experiences that the student will need, so that he or she can meet the aims of the course, which will include some specific learning aims.

A curriculum develops over a long period of time, it is not static and involves all the aspects of setting aims, designing training, delivering training, evaluating, then refining the aims. It is because the curriculum develops as a result of evaluating (assessing) the course that it is learner-centred, and so formative assessment is an essential part of curriculum development. However, a course that is totally learner-centred can be a disaster if the students do not have an overview of their needs, and guidance from a professional who will help them discover what they 'do not know they do not know'. It is one of the course organizer's roles to help with this guidance without allowing the course to become too teacher-centred.

It is unusual to join a course without some kind of curriculum already in place. There is probably no such thing as a perfect curriculum because nothing remains unchanged in medicine, education or our modern world for very long. Change is therefore a powerful stimulus for curriculum development as new aims are needed to meet new challenges. Developing the curriculum is a challenging task that can be quite enjoyable if other course organizers are involved, as is the case on most VTSs. Learners can also be involved and their input helps them develop 'ownership' of their course, meaning that they are more likely to work positively towards achieving the aims of the course, including meeting their own learning needs.

Aims

If the aims are agreed by the organizers of the course, then specific learning objectives can be set and the curriculum will be based on the aims and objectives. A curriculum drawn up without reference to the aims of a course will not be representative of the needs of the course members, and will usually not be good enough to provide the educational input that the organizers planned. It follows that a good curriculum cannot be guaranteed unless aims are set first. The curriculum develops once GP registrars start to understand the concept of learner-centred learning and want to change some aspects of the course. Curriculum development also occurs with changes in the necessary knowledge and skills that will occur with progress. Rather like the audit cycle, curriculum development is continuous and course organizers cannot expect to ignore it for long if they want to have a modern course meeting the learning needs of their GP registrars.

An example of clear aims on which a curriculum was based, together with an example of part of a curriculum, can be found at the end of this chapter.

GP registrar representation

It may seem to most GP registrars, and even many trainers, that the training system is somewhat haphazard and that vocational training in general has developed in a different way in each region. In fact, very clear guidelines about the standards and expectations for a VTS have been laid down by the JCPTGP, just as there are standards identified for the appointment of trainers, from the same committee. Guidelines like these are not set by people without any experience of general practice, or medical education, and as in many areas of education in general practice the professionals involved in the education are consulted. Consultation is generally through a nationwide committee structure whereby regional educational committees, recently renamed educational advisory committees, are able to influence JCPTGP decisions and implement the decisions coming from the JCPTGP. An important aspect of these committees is the GP registrar representation, and there is commonly a GP registrar sub-committee, which has a formal representation on the regional committee. In this way the GP registrar voice can be heard regionally and nationally. This is widely encouraged and time spent working on the sub-committee is seen as extremely valuable by the GP registrars concerned. Representation is by one or two GP registrars from each scheme in a region, with any GP registrar eligible to stand for nomination.

The Royal College of General Practitioners also encourages GP registrar representation, where there is representation on the college council. However, because GP registrars do not usually hold the MRCGP, they are there as observers. This means they are not entitled to vote but they do have the opportunity to speak and their views are listened to and often acted on. There are two GP registrar observers, each standing for 2 years, with one appointed each year so that there is some continuity. Nominations are sought through local college faculties and course organizers, and the only stipulation is that nominees and voters must be associates of the college.

An example of VTS aims

The trainee shall demonstrate his or her ability to:
1 Know what it feels like to be the patient.
2 Maintain the dignity of the patient(s) in all consultations.
3 Practise patient-centred medicine.
4 Identify his or her own learning needs.
5 Remedy his or her own learning needs.
6 Assess himself or herself objectively after learning.
7 Analyse accurately his or her own doctor–patient relationships.
8 Understand illness as deeply in terms of the patient's behaviour as he or she does in terms of the patient's pathology.
9 Assess accurately the capacity of a home/household to care for one of its sick members.
10 Offer, in more than half of an unselected series of consultations in general practice, practical preventive medical advice to his or her patients (opportunistic health promotion; Stott & Davis, 1979).
11 Regard general practice as a branch of medicine in its own right with its own body of knowledge, skills and attitudes.
12 Tolerate uncertainty (McWhinney, 1976).
13 Promote the patient's autonomy.

14 Read and analyse critically the literature of general practice.

15 Regard his or her list of patients as a population at risk for which the doctor is responsible, whether or not they happen to be consulting (McWhinney, 1976).

16 Analyse a problem in medical care, devise a research project to investigate it, gather data, interpret these and write a report of the study.

17 Analyse selected consultations in general practice, using at least three different theoretical models of the consultation in general practice.

18 Manage time efficiently.

19 Work in harmony with colleagues in the medical and nursing professions.

20 Be a good employer.

21 Promote the status and standing of practice nursing within the nursing profession.

22 Foster the development of the role of therapists in primary care.

An example of part of a VTS curriculum

Term 8: Aspects of general practice and human behaviour

- Random-case analysis.
- Problem-case analysis.
- Video-consultation analysis.
- Open and review sessions.
- The practice nurse: teamwork, delegation, autonomy in relationships (joint study afternoon/day with 1-year group).
- Counselling skills.
- Coping with stress.
- GP fundholding.
- Critical journal reading.
- Audit feedback (on audit planned in the previous term and carried out in the meantime).
- Alcoholism/addiction (with 1-year group).
- Models of illness.
- Transactional analysis.
- The use of computers.

Term 9: Nearly there

- Random-case analysis.
- Problem-case analysis.
- Video-consultation analysis.
- Open and review sessions.
- Physiotherapy and the GP.
- Working in teams: problems and successes!
- On being a GP locum.
- Life after the VTS.
- Choosing a practice.
- Book review.

References

Gray, D.J.P. (1977) *Occasional Paper 4—A System of Training for General Practice*. Royal College of General Practitioners, London.

Johnson, D.W. & Johnson, F.P. (1991) *Joining Together*. Prentice Hall, New York.

Knowles, M.S. (1970) *The Modern Practice of Adult Education: From Pedagogy to Androgogy*. Cambridge Book Co., Cambridge.

McWhinney, I.R. (1976) *Department of Family Medicine*. University of Western Ontario, Ontario, Canada.

Pendleton, D., Schofield, T., Tate, P. & Havelock, P. (1984) *The Consultation: an Approach to Learning and Teaching*. Oxford Medical Textbooks, Oxford.

Rogers, A. (1988) *Teaching Adults*. Oxford University Press, Oxford.

Royal College of General Practitioners (1972) *The Future General Practitioner*. RCGP, London.

Stott, N.C.H. & Davis, R.H. (1979) The exceptional potential in each primary care consultation. *Journal of the Royal College of General Practitioners* **29**, 201–205.

Tuckman, B. (1965) Developmental sequence in small groups. *Psychological Bulletin* **63**, 384–399.

7   Preparing for summative assessment

Introduction

Summative assessment was described by John Hasler, in his speech as Chairman of the Conference of UK Advisers, as being one of the great advances in general practice training (J. Hasler, personal communication, 1997). However, a registrar, trying to produce a video tape of satisfactory consultations, may not quite see it that way. Equally, a trainer, struggling to meet the requirements of the regional office, may regard summative assessment as yet another imposition.

This chapter attempts to explain why summative assessment came into being, what is required of GP registrars and trainers and, perhaps most importantly, how to pass the assessment with the minimum of disruption to the training year.

Summative assessment came into force throughout the UK on 4 September 1996. The system of summative assessment currently in use was pioneered in the West of Scotland. In that region all GP registrars completing training after 1 July 1993 took part, and by the autumn of 1997 more than 600 had gone through the system. As a result, a considerable level of experience has been built up in all aspects of summative assessment. Although, at the time of writing, the national situation appears to be stable, all registrars taking part in summative assessment would be advised to check the up-to-date position regarding the details of the process.

Why summative assessment?

Although introduced relatively recently in a formal way, summative assessment has been around for a long time. It has, in fact, developed in parallel with training for general practice and stems from the growing realization that general practice is a specialty in its own right, because the obvious corollary to that realization is that not everyone with a medical degree is by definition a competent GP. The first steps down this road of accreditation took place in 1975, with the formation of the Joint Committee on Postgraduate Training for General Practice (JCPTGP). At that time it was still possible to go straight into general practice after full registration. By 1979 doctors had to complete 1 year as a trainee in general practice to achieve certification, and by 1981 it had become necessary to complete 2 years of approved hospital posts in addition to the trainee year. For all of the posts the trainer had to complete a statement of 'satisfactory completion'. The meaning of satisfactory completion was not clear at the time and it was suggested that it could simply mean completing the appropriate time in the posts. The situation was clarified in 1990 by a statement from the chairmen of the JCPTGP, the General Medical Services Committee and the Royal College of General Practitioners (Irvine *et al.*, 1990), who stated that a doctor entering general practice should have reached an acceptable standard of competence. In effect this was the birth of summative assessment. The only difference from today is that in 1990 it was the sole responsibility of the trainer to make the decision.

It became increasingly clear that all was not well with the system. Studies had shown that many trainers had considered refusing to sign certificates but had continued to sign rather than become involved in a dispute with possible legal consequences. In the mid-1990s there were several high-profile General Medical Council (GMC) cases involving recently certificated doctors, and on at least one occasion a trainer had to appear before the GMC to justify his decision to issue a certificate. By this time the rate of refusal to issue a certificate was running at 0.26%, or around five trainees out of the 2000 a year completing training in the UK. By 1992 there were calls (Carney, 1992) for a national standard for entry into general practice.

The JCPTGP (Joint Committee on Postgraduate Training for General Practice, 1992) set out the basic attributes required in a GP at the end of training (see Box 7.1).

It was clear that no single method would effectively test all of these attributes, and work began to develop a fair system of summative assessment. It was possible, since we were effectively starting with a blank sheet of paper, to try to build certain

---

Box 7.1 Basic attributes required in a GP after training

Adequate:
- knowledge
- problem–solving skills
- clinical competence
- consulting skills
- skills in producing a written report of practical work in general practice
- performance of skills, attitudes and knowledge

Box 7.2 Attributes of the summative assessment programme

- The trainer's assessment should carry weight
- There must be an objective external contribution
- Clinical competence must be directly assessed
- Performance throughout the trainee year should count
- A 100% pass rate should be possible
- The procedure must be feasible

---

desirable attributes into the process. The key attributes are shown in Box 7.2.

Understanding the process will be helped if the importance of these attributes is considered briefly here. The trainer has most opportunity to form a judgement based on the GP registrar's performance over the entire period of training. However, because of the close and friendly relationship that usually develops between the trainer and the registrar during the trainee period, it becomes difficult for the trainer to form an objective and unbiased view of the registrar's performance. Additionally, it could be felt that failure of a trainee to reach a satisfactory level of competence casts doubt on the trainer's ability to appoint an appropriate trainee or provide adequate teaching. The possible conflict of interest is such that an external contribution to the assessment process is necessary to maintain the credibility of the system.

For any assessment method to attain face validity, it must measure an area which is relevant to the eventual professional activities of the candidate. Few would dispute the concept that the main role of the GP is to provide continuing health care for individuals and families. The ability of the doctor to carry out consultations successfully is therefore a major determinant of the doctor's overall competence. It has been shown, for example (Millar & Goldberg, 1991), that GP trainees with good interviewing skills are more likely to offer relevant advice and treatment to patients with psychiatric disorders. Indirect methods of assessing clinical ability can be used, but there is as yet no evidence for a close correlation between these methods and actual clinical competence. There is in fact some evidence that multiple-choice papers and modified essay papers are not by themselves good predictors of postgraduate performance (Rabinowitz, 1987). There appears to be only a modest correlation between performance in written tests and clinical rating scales (Dowaliby & Andrew, 1976).

Individuals have a varying response to the situation of an endpoint exam. There is considerable anecdotal evidence that some candidates do not perform well under exam conditions. Some element of continuous assessment would therefore appear to be desirable.

It would be inappropriate, in an assessment of this nature, to have a built-in failure rate, as occurs in many postgraduate exams. Clearly it should be possible for all candidates to pass. This entails the use of criterion referencing rather than peer referencing, wherever possible. There are obvious difficulties in defining criteria for competence in general practice.

The two possible approaches are to produce a detailed list of attributes or to define competence in broad but imprecise terms —the checklist versus the global approach. For the video component of summative assessment, the global approach was chosen. There is some evidence that such global scales are at least as reliable as more complex marking systems (Millar & Goldberg, 1991).

The final package

It is clear that no single assessment method contains all the important attributes. As a result, the procedure which was ultimately adopted consisted of four distinct but complementary components, which when added together would effectively assess the knowledge, skills and attitudes required for independent practice. The components are shown in Box 7.3.

Box 7.3 Components of the final assessment procedure

- A written paper consisting of multiple true/false and extended matching questions
- A trainer's report
- A submission of written practical work (currently a completed audit).
- Analysis of video-taped consultations

The theoretical background underpinning the individual components is largely beyond the scope of this chapter, but they can be explored further in work reported by Campbell *et al.* (1990, 1993, 1995a,b, 1996a,b,c), Johnson *et al.* (1996a,b: the trainer's report) and Lough *et al.* (1995a,b,c: the audit).

Explanations of the individual elements of the package follow.

The written test of knowledge (MCQ)

Practicalities

The MCQ is available four times a year at regional centres throughout the UK. The dates normally fall on the first Wednesdays in May, September and December, and the second Wednesday in February. Full details of timing and venues are available from your regional director of postgraduate general practice education. There is no charge for sitting the paper and the GP registrars can, if necessary, resit the paper up to three times during the training year. It is theoretically possible to make an attempt at the paper at the first available sitting, but it is recommended that the GP registrars should be in post for at least 3 months before the first attempt.

The scope and nature of the paper

Areas covered by the paper
The questions cover all the areas that are found in general practice. The proportion of questions in each area is shown in Box 7.4.

Box 7.4 Areas covered by the MCQ paper

• Internal medicine (medicine, therapeutics, surgical diagnosis, psychiatry, geriatrics, etc.)—45% of total
• Child health—16.7% of total
• Women's health—16.7% of total
• External medicine (ear, nose and throat, eyes, dermatology)—16.7% of total
• Practice management, etc.—5% of total

The structure of the questions
The paper consists of 300 multiple true/false questions and 20 questions of the extended matching type. Marks are **not** deducted for incorrect answers. Examples of the types of questions asked are given below.

Multiple true/false questions
1 Amenorrhoea may be caused by:
hyperprolactinaemia
premature ovarian failure
rapid weight loss
cessation of the oral contraceptive.
2 Conductive hearing loss is present in:
otosclerosis
infective erosion of the long process of the incus
eustachian tube blockage
cochlear damage.
3 Bulimia is characterized by:
weight fluctuations
laxative abuse
diuretic abuse
marked guilt feelings.
4 L-dopa excess may result in:
hallucinations
vivid dreams
facial dyskinesia
chorea.

5 A footballer presents with an acute knee injury after twisting his leg. Which of the following signs are characteristic of a torn meniscus?
tenderness to palpation over the meniscus
tenderness on deep pressure over the patella locking
retropatellar crepitus on movement of the knee.
6 All children under 10 years of age with urinary tract infection should have:
urine culture and sensitivities
micturating cystourethrogram
intravenous pyelogram
retrograde pyelogram.

Extended matching questions. Select the single most appropriate diagnosis for each of these case histories. A diagnosis may appear more than once or not at all.
1 An 8-year-old boy is brought to the surgery because of peeling skin from his hands and feet. He had been treated with penicillin a week earlier for a mild sore throat. His mother had noticed a transient rash the day after the previous visit.
2 A young man attends with a 3-week history of a reddish-brown rash over his trunk and arms. The lesions started off oval in shape and followed skin cleavage lines. A single similar lesion had appeared a few days before the main crop.

Possible diagnoses for cases 1 and 2:
A allergic rash
B scarlatina
C chickenpox
D tinea versicolor
E measles
F pityriasis rosea
G rubella
H scabies
I glandular fever

Defining the pass mark

In many exams pass marks are determined by working out how many candidates would pass with a given pass mark and then adjusting the pass mark to produce a 'suitable pass rate'. Others use fixed pass marks, for example 50% or 60%, which appear to have no particular justification. In pursuance of the objective that the summative assessment process should identify doctors of minimum acceptable competence, the pass mark is derived using a process which is complicated in its execution but has the simple objective of identifying doctors who have acceptable levels of knowledge. Details of the system used have been reported in papers by Livingstone and Zieky (1982) and De Gruijter (1985), but in essence the systems is as explained below.

A pass mark is derived using the Angof technique, as described by Livingstone and Zieky in 1982. A group of experienced GP principals analyse a section of the question-bank item by item, and for each question produce a figure for the percentage of trainees of minimum acceptable competence whom they would expect to answer the question correctly.

By this means a minimum acceptable overall score is determined. Any candidate scoring below this score fails the exam. The purpose behind using this apparently complex system is to avoid rank ordering, which would result in failure of a predetermined percentage. This runs counter to one of the basic principles of summative assessment: that it should be possible for every trainee to pass the assessment process.

The results

More than 1000 GP registrars have now taken the test, which has been run quarterly throughout the UK since September 1996. The pass mark has usually been in the range 65–70%. The pass rate varies a little, but it is usually around 95%. Bearing in mind that random guessing would result in a score of 50%, it can be seen that to score a pass mark is not onerous. The number of GP registrars not achieving a pass in the three attempts usually available is minimal. However, it is not good for morale to fail the test even at the first attempt, so some preparation is useful.

Preparation

Because most of the material covers the common areas of clinical practice, it is important to be as up to date in the broad range of clinical medicine as possible. It should not be necessary to revise the whole undergraduate curriculum, but it is important to identify areas of potential weakness. Many registrars identify deficiencies in the 'minor' specialties, such as ear, nose and throat, eyes and dermatology, and it would be well worth reading one of the 'ABC' type books covering these fields. Practice tutorials should also be a considerable help, both in identifying areas of need and in addressing them. One of the chief functions of the practice tutorial should be to develop the GP registrars's learning plan by identifying learning needs. The structure and functions of practice tutorials are covered elsewhere, but it is worth emphasizing that tutorials should be discussions between well-informed parties, not a passive transfer of knowledge. The use of a reflective diary by the registrar is highly recommended for identifying and addressing learning needs. This somewhat grandiose expression merely means writing down any gaps in understanding which become apparent during day-to-day work. Writing this down is important—we all identify learning needs during consulting sessions but we tend to 'forget' to do anything about it. How often have you said 'I must look that up', and how often have you actually done it? Writing it down will not ensure that you do look it up, but you will feel even more guilty if you do not. This, of course, applies just as much to trainers as it does to GP registrars.

Specific preparation
It is likely that 'hot' topics will appear in the paper, which tends to be finalized only 3–4 weeks before the exam. It is therefore vital to keep up to date with the journals. A journal review session, involving trainer and trainee or a study group of registrars, will be helpful for both summative assessment and the MRCGP. Box 7.5

Box 7.5 Minimal journal reading throughout the year

* *British Journal of General Practice*—monthly
* *British Medical Journal*—weekly
* An abstract publication, e.g. *Medical Monitor*
* 'The comics'—*GP*, *Pulse*, *Doctor*—for current news

---

contains the minimum journal reading that should be done throughout the year.

Special situations
Most GP registrars will have done the standard collection of SHO jobs after graduating from a UK university in the past 4 years. For those who graduated overseas, who have been in one specialty for a long time or who have limited general experience, there are obviously additional problems. Here identification of learning needs is vital and attachments to hospital clinics for learning/relearning may well be useful.

Specific techniques
There is a remarkable mystique surrounding MCQs, which is mostly quite superfluous. The basic principle is that you will be presented with a statement that is either true or false. Read the question carefully and tick the box you think is most likely to be correct. You may think you do not have a clue, but if you think around the subject a little you may well find that one answer becomes more likely. Because there is no negative marking it is essential to at least attempt each question. There are some basic wording situations to note. If a question includes the words always or never, the answer is guaranteed to be false—as in 'myocardial infarction always presents with chest pain' or 'diabetics never have to pay prescription charges'. Words such as usually, and seldom, characteristically all have their dictionary meanings and should not pose any problems. When percentages are given they will always be right or very wrong, so there is no need to worry about a percentage point here or there. For example, 'meningococcus is the cause of 80% of meningitis in childhood'—this is much too high. Extended matching questions are designed to reward decision-making skills rather than rote learning—because there are many more choices it is obviously harder to guess correctly, but if you think about it carefully the answer should come. Rather than scanning down the list for the most appropriate answer, the best approach is to decide on the answer and then see if your choice is on the list. If it is not a rethink is required.

To summarize, if you start off up to date and keep up to date by reading the journals, the MCQ should pose no problems.

Box 7.6 Requirements for the written submission of practical work

- The work should be the registrar's own; others' work can be used, e.g. for data collection
- Can be done at any time during vocational training, i.e. in hospital jobs
- Must be relevant to general practice
- Must be submitted at least 3 months before the end of training
- Can be resubmitted on two occasions if necessary

The written submission of practical work

At the moment the only acceptable written submission is a completed audit, as developed by Lough *et al.* (1995b). It is likely that other written submissions will be acceptable in the next few years, but it is almost certainly the case that an audit will be acceptable for the foreseeable future. The audit is likely to be the preferred submission by GP registrars for one simple reason. If you carry out and report the audit according to the published protocol, it is almost impossible to fail. Clearly the ability to assess quality of care is important in general practice, but from the point of view of summative assessment the main objective is to test basic audit methods and the GP registrars's objective is likely to be get it out of the way. The practicalities of the audit are shown in Box 7.6.

The marking schedule

To pass, an audit must satisfy all of the following criteria:

Why was the audit done (reason for choice of topic)?
This should be clearly defined and reflected in the title. The audit should have the potential to produce change.

How was the audit done?

Criteria chosen. The criteria should be relevant to the subject of the audit. The criteria should be justified, i.e. evidence-based.

Preparation and planning. This should show the appropriate use of the practice team. The methodology should be satisfactory. Any standards set should be justified.

What was found?—interpretation of data
Relevant data should be used to draw appropriate conclusions.

What next?—detailed proposals for change
Specific proposals to improve the performance of the practice should be produced.

The rough guide to audit success

Some trainers and GP registrars will be audit enthusiasts—many, on the other hand, will be keen to get it out of the way with the minimum expenditure of time and effort. The audit aficionados can skip the next bit. For those remaining, the following is a guide to how to do an audit project with the minimum of fuss.

Pick a topic that has the following characteristics:
• A small, clearly defined clinical area.
• An area where there is a consensus.
• An area involving few patients.
• An area where change should be easy to implement.

Two examples of topics for which audits could be carried out are given below.

Example of a significant event analysis: The lost report (a smear result is not reported to the patient despite being abnormal)
A significant event analysis has the enormous advantage of requiring no data collection and no literature searches. Let us run through the criteria.

Reason for choice. Results should be reported to the patient—this can be potentially disastrous if not. A monitoring system should be practicable.

How was it done:
• Criteria chosen: reports should be acted upon.

- Preparation and planning: should involve explaining to the team what is happening, and seeking ideas on how to deal with the problem.

What was found. Why did the report go missing? Was it an error in the system or an isolated human mistake?

Recommendations for change. How can the system be changed to avoid repetition?

Example of a systematic audit: management of atrial fibrillation

Reasons for choice. There is now a great deal of evidence to support the use of warfarin; a quick literature search should find the papers.

How was it done:
- Criteria chosen: all patients with atrial fibrillation (AF) should be offered warfarin treatment unless there is a specific contraindication.
- Preparation and planning: plan devised to identify all patients with AF after full discussion with the practice team.

What was found. Identify all the patients with AF by computer search, repeat prescribing records, partners' recall, etc. Tabulate the numbers prescribed and not prescribed warfarin, with any reasons for this.

Recommendations for change. It is probable that there are patients who should have been offered warfarin but have not. Devise a system to deal with this and prevent it from happening in the future. For example, call up all the patients with AF and offer them warfarin. Organize a flow chart, to be placed in the records of all newly diagnosed AF patients, which involves raising the issue of warfarin.

Audits as described above should take only a few hours' work and, if done properly, should certainly pass. The types of audits to avoid include complex areas, such as prescribing, large patient populations and a large amount of data to collect. Examples of audits not to carry out include the management of diabetes, asthma or any psychological areas. Also be sure to avoid areas where there is no proven benefit, for example exercise in pregnancy or attendance at counselling.

The video

The video is seen by most trainers and GP registrars as the most threatening component of summative assessment. It certainly produces the highest failure rate. However, provided the GP registrar can consult effectively, it should be relatively straightforward to succeed.

Technical requirements

The practical requirements should be dealt with first and these are shown in Box 7.7.

The following points should be borne in mind.

Many practices use camcorders which record on small-format tape. These tapes are easily transcribed to standard VHS. The training practice should have the facilities to do this. It is unacceptable to run into problems every year. Once the equipment is organized, there should really be no further problem. Camera positioning is important. A wall bracket is often useful for locating the camera. The built-in microphones supplied with camcorders are often inadequate, and an additional desk-top or directional microphone is often necessary to produce adequate sound quality. It is important to remember that video assessors are likely to be older than GP registrars, with the consequent reduction in hearing acuity that

---

Box 7.7 Practical requirements for video submission

- The tape must be at least 2 hours long
- Informed written consent from patients must be obtained
- The tape submitted should be a standard VHS tape
- The picture should show both the GP registrar and patient
- The sound must be of acceptable quality
- The tape should be time/date-stamped
- The consultation log must be completed

age brings. In addition, it's worth remembering that, although the assessors will try to comprehend the content of a poor-quality tape, there is no guarantee that they will not miss things.

The marking system

Although a marking schedule is used by the assessors to help them come to a judgement, there is no scoring system. Therefore the final decision is based on the assessors' overall judgement of the competence displayed on the material submitted. The criteria used by the assessors are discussed fully below.

Listening

The GP registrar should identify and elucidate the reason(s) for the patient's attendance. Negotiation of acceptable management plans should take place.

Action

The GP registrar should take appropriate action to identify the patient's problem(s). Investigations and referrals should be reasonable. Help should be sought when necessary. The patient's problem should be managed appropriately.

Understanding

The GP registrars should demonstrate in the logbook that he or she understands the process and the outcome of the consultation. Individual actions should be explained. Obvious shortcomings in the consultation should be identified. Relevant background information should be mentioned.

Errors

If a major error or a series of minor errors in patient management is noted, the GP registrar may be referred. A major error is defined as one that causes actual or potential harm; a minor error causes inconvenience only.

The referral process

The referral process is shown diagrammatically in Fig. 7.1.

The system is designed to produce consistent and fair results

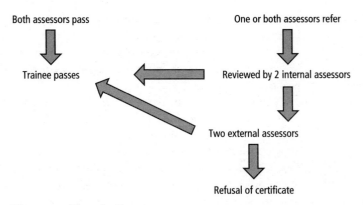

Figure 7.1 The referral process.

across the country with the maximum of reliability. Each tape is first seen independently by two assessors within the region. They are asked to refer on any trainee about whom they have any doubts and they are encouraged to refer if they have the slightest doubt about the acceptability of the GP registrar. This aspect of the process is designed to maximize sensitivity, i.e. to ensure that no unsatisfactory GP registrars get through. If either or both of these assessors refer, the tape is then reviewed by two second-level assessors within the region. These assessors work together and are asked to determine if the GP registrar's performance is poor enough to justify the need for further training. If they decide that the performance is adequate, the trainee passes. If, on the other hand, the second-level assessors think that retraining is required, the tape is referred on to two assessors randomly selected from a national panel. These assessors review the tape and the written comments of the first- and second-level assessors. Once again, if they think the trainee is acceptable, the GP registrar passes; if they agree with the verdict of the second-level assessors, the GP registrar will be recommended for a further 6 months of training with a resubmission at that time.

What and when to submit

Although the level of performance required is not high, it is important to ensure that the tape submitted represents a true reflection of the performance of the GP registrar. It should not be necessary to submit a greatest-hits collection. Provided the registrar is competent in consulting, a straightforward tape of normal consultations should be enough, but there are several points to bear in mind.

Competence has to be demonstrated—therefore the tape must contain some consultations requiring consulting skills. Most consultations do require some skills but it would be wise to avoid consultations with no challenge. For example, a patient attending for a note to return to work after a minor operation or a routine blood-pressure check in a patient with well-controlled high blood pressure is unlikely to enable the GP registrar to demonstrate competence.

Many GP registrars submit long consultations that contain very little meat but a lot of social chit-chat. Once again, such a consultation is unlikely to enable the GP registrar to demonstrate competence and should be avoided.

One of the major questions is whether to edit out a consultation that has gone wrong. If a serious error has been committed, it would be unwise to submit that consultation.

The tape must be submitted no later than 3 months before the end of training, because it can take 3 months to get a result. Most regions insist that the GP registrar waits at least 6 months after commencing training before submitting the tape. Normally only one submission is allowed during the training year and, if the tape fails, a further 6 months of training is recommended.

Is the tape good enough?
The GP registrar should not submit a tape without it being reviewed by the trainer in the practice. The trainer is unlikely to be a trained assessor, and in any event the close relationship between trainer and GP registrar may well make objectivity impossible. However, the trainer should at least try to ensure that the material on the tape is a true reflection of the GP registrar's normal performance. The regular use of video tapes for formative assessment should enable problems to be identified early and dealt with. There is no point in coaching in this context, but if the GP registrar has mastered the appropriate consulting skills the tape should not be a problem.

Common characteristics of tapes which fail
No two GP registrars consult in an identical fashion and that is a good thing. However, a large proportion of failing tapes do have certain characteristics in common, and it is worth bearing these in mind when assessing if a tape is suitable for submission.

1 Listening.
- The doctor interrupts early in the consultation.
- Closed questions appear early on.
- Solutions are offered before problems are properly identified.
- Potentially significant symptoms are not explored.

2 Action.
- Patients are referred often and inappropriately.
- A rational management plan is not developed.
- A prescription is offered as a reflex solution to every problem—symptom swatting.
- Management can seem extremely idiosyncratic.
- Follow-up arrangements are unclear.

3 Understanding.
- The doctor's description does not match the consultation.
- Data are missing: for example, prescriptions.
- There is a lot of *post hoc* rationalization; for example, 'I'll deal with this next week.'

The log

Filling in the log should be very straightforward. It is important to give the appropriate information; for example, if an antibiotic has been prescribed it should be specified which one was used, or if there were clinical findings on examination these should be noted. If a mistake has been made or a consultation went wrong, it is important to acknowledge this in the log. However, a series of poor consultations with log diaries full of insight and explanation is not likely to result in a pass.

The structured trainer's report
This report has been developed by Neil Johnson in the Oxford region and details of the thinking behind it can be found in several published papers (Johnson *et al.*, 1996a,b). It contains a checklist of attributes that the trainer is asked to verify (see Box 7.8).

Box 7.8 Checklist of attributes for trainer to verify

- General clinical skills—such as problem recognition, knowledge, diagnostic skills
- Clinical judgement—examination, investigations
- Communication skills
- Personal and professional growth—can identify own strengths and weaknesses
- Organizational skills—time management
- Professional values—ethics, responsibility
- Specific clinical skills

Completing the log

The best way to deal with the log is to refer to it early in training and to complete sections as training proceeds. If this is done, there should be no last-minute rush to check things out and by sharing doubts with the registrar at an early stage it should be possible to at least address potential difficulties before it becomes too late. The golden rule is that there should be enough feedback during training to ensure that the result of the trainer's report comes as no surprise to any GP registrar. From a trainer's point of view it is important to realize that the report is a formal document for which the trainer could be held accountable.

Problems with the log

The main difficulty is that the trainer is asked to record some skills which most of us would assume had been learned adequately at undergraduate level: for example, taking a blood pressure, doing a rectal examination. However, it is important that the trainer has good grounds for stating that the GP registrar can carry out these activities. This problem can be dealt with in several ways. For example, registrars in many specialties keep a logbook in which practical procedures are recorded. This could be used as the basis for completing the log. Many regions now have clinical skills laboratories, and it would be possible for the registrar to attend an assessment to obtain evidence of competence in practical procedures.

Box 7.9 Pass and failure rates: West of Scotland

Total number	603
Failed video	23
Failed trainer's report	7 (2 failed video)
Failed audit	1 (also failed report)
Failed MCQ	0
Total passes	575 (95.4%)

The overall results

A major concern for many trainers and GP registrars will be the likelihood of failure. The system has been running since 1993 in the West of Scotland and data are now available on more than 600 GP registrars who have gone through the system. The early results for the UK are similar to the West of Scotland data. It is important to remember that all components must be passed. Doing well in one will not compensate for failing another. The overall pass rates up until the end of 1997 for the West of Scotland and the contribution of the individual components are shown in Box 7.9.

This box shows that the video is the main cause of failure and that the audit and MCQ produce very few failures. The overall fail rate is currently just under 5%, but it is important to realize that this will vary from year to year because of the criterion-based way in which the programme works.

The workload for the year

One of the major complaints from trainers and GP registrars is that the trainee year is now severely overcrowded. Certainly it is true that it is no longer a year which GP registrars can treat as a holiday after the hard work of hospital posts. But it should never have been a holiday anyway. The value of the hospital posts is pretty dubious much of the time and the real learning is carried out in the general practice year. It is to be hoped that the pilot schemes in which 18 months are spent in practice will eventually develop to become the norm. This will take much of the pressure off the trainee year.

Box 7.10 Plan for completing all elements of summative assessment

1 Start doing formative video at the beginning of the year
2 Start thinking about the audit project in the first couple of months
3 Read the journals and deal with educational needs as you go along
4 Sit the MCQ 6 months into the year
5 Complete the video and the audit by the 8th month
6 Complete the trainer's report as the occasion arises throughout the year

---

Planning

The most common mistake that GP registrars make is to put off doing the elements of summative assessment until the last minute. This produces anxiety and unnecessary pressure. It is astonishing how often regional offices are phoned by GP registrars seeking an extension to the deadline for handing in the video because, for example, 'the person who works the video is on holiday', 'the video sound wasn't switched on', 'the dog ate the video', etc. Such behaviour is hardly professional and is unlikely to produce acceptable work. The plan shown in Box 7.10 is suggested to avoid the last-minute panic.

Summative assessment and the MRCGP examination

It is highly likely that passing the MRCGP examination will, in due course, provide exemption from all of summative assessment except the trainer's report. All that is needed is for the college to demonstrate that the exam is as effective as summative assessment at identifying the GP registrar who is not at an acceptable level of competence. It is already possible to use the exam MCQ as an exemption and the same video tape for both assessments. However, it would be an unwise GP registrar who took the exemption route. Summative assessment requires the same kind of preparation as the exam, it can be taken at no cost to the GP registrar and it has a much lower failure rate than the MRCGP exam. For these reasons most registrars who sit the MRCGP exam would be well advised to use summative assessment as an insurance policy against failing one of the MRCGP components.

References

Campbell, L.M. & Murray, T.S. (1990) Trainee assessment—a regional survey. *British Journal of General Practice* **40**, 507–509.

Campbell, L.M. & Murray, T.S. (1996a) Assessment of competence. *British Journal of General Practice* **46**, 619–622.

Campbell, L.M. & Murray, T.S. (1996b) Summative assessment of vocational trainees: results of a 3-year study. *British Journal of General Practice* **46**, 411–414.

Campbell, L.M. & Murray, T.S. (1996c) The effects of the introduction of a system of mandatory formative assessment for general practice trainees. *Medical Education* **30**, 60–64.

Campbell, L.M., Howie, J.G. & Murray, T.S. (1993) Summative assessment: a pilot project in the west of Scotland. *British Journal of General Practice* **43**, 430–434.

Campbell, L.M., Howie, J.G. & Murray, T.S. (1995a) Use of videotaped consultations in summative assessment of trainees in general practice. *British Journal of General Practice* **45**, 137–141.

Campbell, L.M., Sullivan, F. & Murray, T.S. (1995b) Videotaping of general practice consultations: effect on patient satisfaction. *British Medical Journal* **311**, 236.

Carney, T. (1992) A national standard for entry into general practice. *British Medical Journal* **305**, 1449–1450.

De Gruijter, D.N.M. (1985) Compromise models for establishing examination standards. *Journal of Educational Measurement* **22**, 263–266.

Dowaliby, F.J. & Andrew, B.J. (1976) Relationships between clinical competence ratings and examination performance. *Journal of Medical Education* **51**, 181–188.

Irvine, D.H., Gray, D.J.P. & Bogle, I.G. (1990) Vocational training for general practice: the meaning of 'satisfactory completion' [letter]. *British Journal of General Practice* **40**, 434.

Johnson, N., Hasler, J., Toby, J. & Grant, J. (1996a) Consensus minimum standards for use in a trainer's report for summative assessment in general practice. *British Journal of General Practice* **46**, 140–144.

Johnson, N., Hasler, J., Toby, J. & Grant, J. (1996b) Content of a trainer's report for summative assessment in general practice: views of trainers. *British Journal of General Practice* **46**, 135–139.

Joint Committee on Postgraduate Training for General Practice (1992) *Report of the Working Party on Summative Assessment.* RCGP, London.

Livingstone, S.A. & Zieky, M.J. (1982) *Passing Scores.* Educational Testing Service, Princeton, New Jersey.

Lough, J.R., McKay, J. & Murray, T.S. (1995a) Audit and summative assessment: a criterion-referenced marking schedule. *British Journal of General Practice* **45**, 607–609.

Lough, J.R., McKay, J. & Murray, T.S. (1995b) Audit and summative assessment: two years' pilot experience. *Medical Education* **29**, 101–103.

Lough, J.R., McKay, J. & Murray, T.S. (1995c) Audit: trainers' and trainees' attitudes and experiences. *Medical Education* **29**, 85–90.

Millar, T. & Goldberg, D.P. (1991) Links between the ability to detect and manage emotional disorders. A study of general practitioner trainees. *British Journal of General Practice* **41**, 257–259.

Rabinowitz, H.K. (1987) The modified essay question: an evaluation of its use in a family medicine clerkship. *Medical Education* **21**, 114–118.

8 The MRCGP

Background

When the Royal College of General Practitioners (RCGP) was formed, members were admitted simply by the payment of a membership fee. The first five candidates took the MRCGP examination in 1965, and in 1968 it became a requirement for membership. The standard represented that expected of a GP aspiring to be a member of the college, or, more informally, was the candidate professionally suitable to join the 'club'?

The early candidates were mainly experienced practitioners. It has now become a test of good practice at the end of vocational training and it is usual to take the examination towards the end of vocational training, or in the early years of practice. It has also become a requirement for career development in fields such as general practice education. Consequently experienced doctors, such as 'would-be trainers', are taking the examination alongside GP registrars. In taking an examination set at 'end-of-training' level, they have to work harder on the knowledge-based parts of the examination, but often excel in other parts where their experience helps in thinking through context-based problems.

The move to modularization

The examination is respected within and outside the profession, in the UK and around the world, as a well-researched, high-quality examination. This has been achieved by a policy of continued review and development.

The panel of examiners is made up of working GPs from all over the UK. They meet formally every year to review the development of the examination, led by the convenor of the panel, and guided by the examination board of the college, where the policies of college council are integrated with the examination organization. The examination regularly draws on the advice of its retained consultants in examination methods. A policy of external review has helped to bring fresh thinking. Experts have been commissioned to advise on its development, and have included teams from America, Dundee and Cambridge.

The MRCGP examination has recognized its role not just in assessing individual doctor's standards, but also in responding to educational needs. For example, the examiners recognized that examinees found it difficult to critically appraise the available literature, and make their own decisions about management based on the evidence rather than the views of an expert in secondary care. As a result, the critical reading paper was developed.

This policy of continued review has made the examination increasingly reliable and more relevant. The cost of the search for excellence was, however, that each new idea became an additional part. The consequence was a rather large examination, which was becoming daunting to many trainers and GP registrars. This arose at the same time as the introduction of Summative Assessment, thus making the GP registrar year even more pressurized.

The solution has been to try and simplify it by a process of modularization and 'credit accumulation'. MRCGP is awarded when a candidate has achieved a pass in each of the modules and met the other membership requirements.

This modular approach gives the potential to link with other assessments. The college is developing an alternative route to membership, 'membership by assessment of performance (MAP)', based on an assessment of the practitioner in the workplace. MAP and the MRCGP examination might overlap in using modules such as the consulting skills component. An MRCGP international could be developed, using some of the current modules and some specially designed. Other professional activities might recognize passes in individual modules. The modular system will also allow the examination to adapt to the ever-changing syllabus.

Examination structure

The examination consists of four modules based around different testing methods and a precertification requirement in child health surveillance and resuscitation (see Table 8.1).

Table 8.1 Modules of the MRCGP.

Module	Components rested
Paper 1: written paper	All that is best tested in prose form
Paper 2: machine-marked paper	All that is best tested in machine-marked format
Consulting skills (video/simulated surgery)	All that is best tested by direct observation
Orals	All that is best tested by structured dialogue with an examiner

The modules stand alone, and can be taken all at once or in any order. When all modules are passed, the MRCGP is awarded. Candidates may start at any stage of their vocational training, and have 3 years from their initial application to complete the examination. Each module is offered twice a year, and each module can be resat twice on payment of a resit fee.

The successful candidates in each module will be awarded either a pass or, for the top 25% or so, a pass with merit. Those passing the examination overall and receiving a merit in two modules are awarded MRCGP with merit, and those receiving a merit in three or four papers are awarded MRCGP with distinction.

Hopefully the prospect of receiving merits will encourage candidates to work for a high standard, and not just a pass.

The syllabus

The syllabus sounds daunting, and includes the knowledge, skills and attitudes that are relevant to the profession of general practice in the context of UK health care. The syllabus is constantly changing, and the new modular system should enable the examination to take on changes without having to enlarge. The modules are based around testing methods rather than topics, so, when a new topic is recognized as important, it can be incorporated into the most appropriate part.

Box 8.1   The blueprint: domains

1 Factual knowledge
2 Evolving knowledge: uncertainty, 'hot topics', qualitative research
3 The evidence base of practice: knowledge of literature, quantitative research
4 Critical appraisal skills: interpretation of literature, principles of statistics
5 Application of knowledge: justification, prioritizing, audit
6 Problem solving: general applications
7 Problem solving: case-specific, clinical management
8 Personal care: matching principles to individual patients
9 Written communication
10 Verbal communication: the consultation process
11 The practice context: 'team' issues, practice management, business skills
12 Regulatory framework of practice (e.g. legal, medicopolitical)
13 The wider context: medicopolitical, legal and societal issues
14 Ethnic and transcultural issues
15 Values and attitudes: ethics, integrity, consistency, *caritas*
16 Self-awareness: insight, reflective learning, 'the doctor as a person'
17 Commitments to maintaining standards: personal and professional growth, continuing medical education

(From MRCGP Examination Regulations (Royal College of General Practitioners, 1998))

In order to ensure that areas of the syllabus are tested in the most appropriate parts, a process of blueprinting (which describes areas of the syllabus and the apportionment of them to parts of the examination) has been undertaken and is regularly reviewed. The blueprint consists of domains—generalizable skills, attributes and competencies, and contexts.

Box 8.1 lists the domains and Table 8.2 shows where each domain is most likely to be tested. Within each module the relevant domains are tested in a variety of contexts. Examples are given in Box 8.2.

Table 8.2 Where the domains are tested.

Module	Domains
Paper 1	1 2 3 4 5 6 7 8 9 (10) 11 13 14 16
Paper 2	1 2 3 (4) 7 12 14
Consulting skills	7 8 10 (15)
Oral	4 5 6 (7) 8 10 11 13 (14) 15 16 17

From MRCGP Examination Regulations (Royal College of General
Practitioners, 1998).
Domains shown in parentheses have only occasional or partial relevance to
the module.

Box 8.2 The blueprint: contexts

The doctor as:
- clinician
- family physician
- patient's advocate
- gatekeeper
- resource allocator
- handler of information
- team member
- team leader
- partner
- colleague
- employer
- manager
- business person
- learner
- teacher
- reflective practitioner
- researcher
- agent and shaper of social policy
- member of a profession
- person and individual

General preparation

The initial feeling of many candidates when starting preparation for the MRCGP is horror at the vastness of the syllabus. Anything could come up, and, from looking at past papers, it often does! This is no different from everyday general practice. We never know what problem the next patient will present. Living with uncertainty is part of the excitement and challenge of general practice.

When we look more closely, things are slightly more predictable. Common things are common, in life and the MRCGP. Topical issues for candidates and their patients are topical for the examiners. The principles of problem solving used in one situation will apply in others, even though the context and specific problem have changed.

In considering how to prepare, consider the examiners' aim. It is to try to promote and assess good general practice. The examiner will judge a candidate's management as if he or she had experienced that consultation, as an informed patient, on a good day, but allowing for the realities of time constraints. The best preparation for the MRCGP is undoubtedly to see patients, go to practice meetings, reflect on and talk about what is seen and experienced, read around problems encountered and about topical issues. Many readers will remember the 'pill scare' of 1995, when many doctors awoke one morning to news in the press that some of the combined oral contraceptive pills containing newer progestogens were reported as having a higher risk of serious side effects. Without any prior warning, GPs had to cope with a flood of enquiries from worried patients. At an oral examination a few weeks later, a candidate was asked how she would have responded to a patient in that situation, worried about the risks. The reply was that she had no idea. She had not taken any interest in the issue as she was too busy revising for the MRCGP!

So is there any difference in preparing for the examination as well as for a life in practice? I believe there are no important differences, just some additional considerations.

The MRCGP is an examination, and therefore inevitably an artificial context. It is well worth getting acquainted with the format by spending time working through old papers. The most effective way to do this is to form a small group with other candidates. Study old papers together, try out oral questions on each other and look at each other's videos. Compare individual performances with that of the group. A small group of candidates collectively will almost invariably cover the same areas in their answers as the examiners.

Paper 1: the written paper

Paper 1 is a 3-hour written paper, usually with 12 or more questions. There is additional time, typically 30 minutes, for reading presented material that usually appertains to the critical appraisal questions.

The content of the answer, rather than its length, attracts marks. The aim is to communicate understanding of the issues to the examiner. Short notes are acceptable unless otherwise instructed. The paper consists of a combined question and answer page for each question. These are sent to different examiners, so avoid making references in one question to previous answers.

It is important to read the questions carefully, and answer the question posed. This should be obvious, but in the heat of the examination it is easy to misread the question and answer a different one. Time management is crucial. It is hard to perform well if questions are left out altogether. It is easier to get the first few marks in a question than the last few.

There have traditionally been four question types and these are described in detail below. More recently, questions have been developed to link knowledge of current literature, and critical appraisal, to critical problem solving.

1. Questions designed to test knowledge and interpretation of general practice literature

These questions are much feared by candidates; there seems to be so much published! The examiners are also working GPs and selective in what they read. Concentrate on:

- Editorials and papers in mainstream journals relevant to general practice, such as the *British Medical Journal* and the *British Journal of General Practice*.
- Articles in *Bandolier* and magazines such as *The Practitioner* and *Update*.

- Papers relevant to everyday general practice, i.e. on topics which are common, chronic and important.
- Topical issues about which there have been several papers, or some controversy.
- Issues where there has been evidence that should make us rethink our management.
- Older papers where these are 'classics' that have changed practice.
- RCGP occasional papers.
- Guidelines of national status.
- Major systematic reviews: *Evidence-based Medicine* journal.
- Do not forget the book literature of general practice.

These questions are not about memorizing references, but about understanding the way literature influences practice. You can pass a question by understanding and presenting the views that have been expressed around the subject without quoting the source. The better candidate may be able to quote specific papers and give a summary of the conclusions, or a brief critical appraisal.

In preparation make your own brief summaries of important papers. Opportunities in tutorials or peer-group meetings to discuss and debate the literature on relevant topics help you to assimilate the relevant concepts and hear about papers you may have missed. Keep notes on patients seen in surgery and searching for literature that can help with their management. Groups of peers working together can share the work of finding relevant papers and pool their findings. Copies of papers can be organized and summarized under topic headings. Least useful is the trainer finding all the papers for the GP registrar. Much of the learning comes from finding papers for oneself, and they are rarely memorable if copied and handed out by a trainer (see Box 8.3).

Box 8.3 Preparing for the knowledge of literature questions

- Study the papers around topics rather than just reading past issues of journals
- Read around problems encountered in practice
- Understand the key messages and appraise the quality of the papers, rather than memorizing lists of references
- Concentrate on articles that have influenced the way we practise

2. Questions testing the ability to evaluate and interpret written material which is presented

In these questions the candidate is presented with short pieces of written material. These may be extracts from papers, such as a methods section, or a summary. The candidate will be expected to interpret any results, and to understand simple statistical ideas, such as confidence intervals, odds ratios, numbers needed to treat, predictive values, sensitivity and specificity. You may be asked to use the information given, after critical consideration, to manage a clinical scenario. Other types of written material may be presented, such as referral letters, memoranda from directors of public health and drug company advertising.

The temptation when reading papers is to go first to the summary and discussion and spend little time on the methods. There is then the danger of changing your practice on the basis of poor or irrelevant research. Critical appraisal teaches us to assess the methods and results to find out if the results are likely to be valid, what they really mean and whether they can be generalized to one's own patients.

In preparing for the examination, and future practice, get into the habit of briefly appraising any paper you read. Look at the methods and results section first. If these are satisfactory read on. If not, do not waste your time.

Refer to Box 8.4 for further guidance on answering these questions.

Box 8.4 Critical appraisal reading list

Useful sources of help with these questions are the excellent series of articles published in the 'Education and Debate' section of the *British Medical Journal* in 1997 by Trisha Greenhalgh and colleagues, and the series of articles published by David Sackett and colleagues in the *Journal of the American Medical Association* (starting with Oxman *et al.*, 1993). The magazine *Bandolier* has occasional articles on understanding and using simple statistical ideas, written for the interested novice. Four excellent books are *Evidence-based Medicine—How to Practice and Teach EBM* by D. L. Sackett *et al.*, *Clinical Epidemiology —A Basic Science for Clinical Medicine* by D. L. Sackett *et al.*, *Critical Reading for the Reflective Practitioner* by R. Clarke and P. Croft, and *Evidence-based General Practice* by L. Ridsdale (see Further reading).

3. Questions testing the ability to integrate and apply theoretical knowledge and professional values to practical problems encountered in an NHS setting

These questions look at the challenges of everyday general practice, where often the evidence is not there to guide us in our decision making or, even if it is, there are many other factors to take into account. They will cover individual patient care, the practice team and its management and wider social, political and ethical issues. Some of the broad topic areas are given in Box 8.5.

Box 8.5 Problem-solving topic areas

- Skills in problem solving, prioritizing and decision making in a wide range of clinical settings
- Insight into the psychological processes affecting the patient, the doctor and the relationship between them
- Recognition of the family, social, occupational, environmental and cultural contexts of ill health
- Communication and consultation skills
- Understanding the principles of preventive medicine and the promotion of good health
- Attitude to patients, colleagues and staff
- Appropriate use of resources, including drugs, treatment facilities, referral agencies, other members of the health-care team, ancillary staff and complementary practitioners
- Appreciation of ethical principles and the GP's terms of service
- Awareness of current or foreseeable trends and developments in primary care

(See RCGP World Wide Web page)

There appear to be two different types of problem-solving situation. One involves sequential 'logical-deductive' thought. An example from a past paper would be:

> Lisa, a girl of three, attends for follow-up after a bout of abdominal pain and fever. A mid-stream specimen of urine has shown a heavy growth of *E. coli* and more than 50 white blood cells per field. Discuss your investigation and management.

Other questions require a much more 'lateral-thinking' approach. An example might be question 12 in the October 1995 paper:

> Books offering advice to GPs include the following:
> 'Make diagnoses in physical, psychological and social terms', and 'Explore the patient's ideas, concerns and expectations'. What do you think of such advice?

Both types of problem solving are relevant to the challenges of practice, and, although the contexts and situations will change between papers, the principles and methods are generally similar. The more a GP registrar practises solving problems, in the practice, in the consulting room and working through old papers, the easier it will be to solve apparently new problems. Experience combined with curiosity and reflection is the key to preparation.

Many candidates worry about the **constructs** used in the marking schedules, as if guessing these would lead to success in answering questions. Constructs are the important themes in a question, and marks are allocated according to performance on each construct. They are called constructs rather than themes for the purpose of examination marking in that they aim to be **singular** and **independent**. The simple reason for this is that it would be unfair on a candidate to mark two themes that overlap. If a candidate thought of one, he or she would be bound to think of the other and hence score marks twice for the same idea or, even worse, leave them out and lose marks twice. An example might be how to decide on the management of a patient with a sore throat. The history, examination and investigations could all be considered separate themes, but in most candidates' minds they are linked—if you think of one, you will probably think of the others—so they might be combined into one construct called clinical issues. On the other hand, the issue of the evidence for and against using antibiotics to treat a sore throat is a separate construct, singular and independent relative to the clinical issues. The constructs are a device to help the examiners and are best ignored by candidates. Remember, in marking the questions the examiners are asking themselves the question 'if I were an informed patient, how would I judge the quality of that consultation?' They are not asking if the candidate has guessed the constructs.

There is no 'negative marking' in paper 1, but candidates can do worse by writing more and exposing their ignorance. One candidate in a question involving advice on holiday travel listed every known inoculation, including smallpox and MMR, perhaps hoping to get marks on the basis of 'ticks' for the correct ones and no marks for the wrong ones! The examiners, however, were looking for a good consultation, and 15 injections, most of them unnecessary, did not impress.

The aim in the answers should be to communicate the ideas clearly and concisely to the examiner. How a candidate does this is up to them. The examiners will be happy with short notes, rambling prose, diagrams, verse or whatever communicates effectively. A good way to ensure that the examiner knows that the candidate really understands what is meant is to illustrate it with an example. Rather than just say that there might be underlying anxieties, one might speculate at what these might be from the context of the question.

Other examination techniques have been proposed elsewhere. A favourite is to look at each question and see how it fits into preordained frameworks, such as 'physical, psychological and social', or the 'patient, doctor, practice, NHS, society, etc.'. These frameworks can be useful when they correlate with how you would solve the problem in real life. However, real-life problems do not conveniently fit into frameworks, and basing answers on them risks leaving out important themes. It is usually best to answer a question by thinking about it as you would if encountering it in practice. If a framework then helps to avoid missing something or someone, then use it, but only as an adjunct.

It is important to communicate effectively with the examiner. Sometimes what may seem obvious to one person is not to another. The examiner can only give credit for that which is written down. Learning to describe clearly what one does is also a valuable skill for continued reflective learning. There is a parallel in how the police rapid response drivers are trained. They already have considerable driving experience, but some bad habits. They are asked to drive with an instructor present, and at the same time describe what they are doing from moment to moment. In doing this they bring subconscious skills back to the surface, and can thus review them. In the context of general practice this is

> **Box 8.6** Skills used by the good candidate
>
> The good candidate:
> - Reads each question carefully, and answers it as asked
> - Thinks in a wide-ranging way, but realistically, about how a competent and sensitive GP would deal with each scenario
> - Avoids jargon, clichés and overgeneralization
> - Includes illustrative details, explanations and relevant examples
>
> (See RCGP World Wide Web page)

important, both to communicate what you do to the examiners and also to help future learning (see Box 8.6).

4. New question formats

These may include:
- Topical questions, which may be not set up until a week or two before the examination.
- Questions combining problem solving with an understanding of current evidence or critical appraisal.
- Short structured answers. The candidate is given a structure for the answer, for example listing the evidence on one side with some details of the source, strength and reliability on the other. These help the candidate to focus their answer. A pass mark can still be obtaining by just knowing and understanding the evidence. The better candidates will offer some details of the source and its quality.

Paper 2: the machine-marked paper

Paper 2 is a 3-hour paper of machine-marked items. There are two sections. One section contains multiple-choice questions (MCQs), either of the true/false type, or select the single best answer to the question from a choice of possible answers. There may be up to 400 true/false items. The other section contains extended matching questions (EMQs), which give an opportunity to test knowledge in a relevant context. These typically consist of situations that have to be matched to answers from a list of options. For each question the candidate has to choose the one best option. A given option may be the answer to more than one question, and some options may not be answers to any of the questions. The EMQs may include graphs, charts and photographs; for example, an ECG reading or a photograph of a skin rash. There are up to 50 EMQs.

In all questions there is one mark for a correct answer and none for a wrong answer. It is strongly recommended to have a go at all the questions. The aim is to test pure and applied knowledge, not confidence.

A great deal of care goes into avoiding ambiguity in the questions. Each paper consists of a mixture of old and new questions. Questions are statistically tested for reliability before the marks are calculated. Marks for a question which is unreliable will be excluded from the final marks. A question is considered reliable when it discriminates in such a way that the people who do well in that question also do better in Paper 2 overall.

Questions are derived from review articles and original papers in journals relevant to general practice. Important sources include:
- *British Medical Journal.*
- *British Journal of General Practice.*
- *Evidence-based Medicine.*
- *Drugs and Therapeutics Bulletin.*
- *Bandolier.*

There is a preponderance of questions on general medicine. The other topic areas occur in roughly equal proportions. Questions are mixed up within the paper (see Box 8.7).

The questions should be unambiguous. To help clarify the meaning of the questions, Box 8.8 gives the definition of commonly used terms.

Preparation for Paper 2 requires a reflective approach to patients seen and problems encountered in practice, looking up the relevant information in books and journals. The candidate should keep up to date with the journals listed above, particularly with regard to topical areas and those relevant to general practice. Several books and magazine columns contain MCQs and EMQs that are valuable for practice. Some, however, are not representative of the current format and have ambiguous questions.

Box 8.7 Paper 2: topic areas

- Critical appraisal, including knowledge of statistics and research methodology sufficient to evaluate published papers
- Current literature
- General medicine and surgery
- Medical specialties, e.g. dermatology, ophthalmology, ear, nose and throat
- Women's health
- Child health
- Service management

(Adapted from Membership Examination Regulations (Royal College of General Practitioners, 1998))

Box 8.8 Common terms in Paper 2

- **Pathognomonic**, **Diagnostic**, **Characteristic** and **In the vast majority** imply a feature would occur in at least 90% of cases
- **Typically**, **Frequently**, **Significantly**, **Commonly** and **In a substantial majority** imply that a feature would occur in greater than 60% of cases
- **In the majority** implies that a feature occurs in greater than 50% of cases
- **In the minority** implies that a feature occurs in less than 50% of cases
- **Low chance** and **In a substantial minority** imply that a feature may occur in up to 30% of cases
- **Has been shown, Recognized** and **Reported** all refer to evidence which can be found in an authoritative medical text. None of these terms makes any implication about the frequency with which the feature occurs

(From Membership Examination Regulations (Royal College of General Practitioners, 1998))

More questions on critical appraisal, current literature, statistics, epidemiology and research design are now set than previously. The examiners are mainly testing the key messages from papers, and the evidence upon which everyday clinical decisions are made.

Examples of questions in Paper 2

True/false MCQs
Recognized causes of haemoptysis include:
  Mitral incompetence
  false
  Upper respiratory tract infection
  true
  Acute left ventricular failure
  false
  Uncomplicated asbestosis
  false
  Sarcoidosis
  false

Single best answer MCQ
In the management of croup in a 2-year-old child, which single treatment has been shown in clinical trials to shorten the course of the condition?:
  place the child in a steam-filled room
  administer inhaled budesonide ★
  prescribe amoxycillin 125 mg t.d.s. for 5 days
  prescribe a paediatric cough suppressant containing codeine
  administer inhaled tribavirin.

★ is correct.

EMQ
Theme: Reduced vision in the eye
Option list:
A   basilar migraine
B   cerebral tumour
C   cranial arteritis
D   macular degeneration
E   occlusion of the central retinal artery
F   occlusion of the central retinal vein
G   demyelinating optic neuritis
H   retinal detachment
I   tobacco optic neuropathy

Instructions: For each patient with reduced vision, select the most likely diagnosis. Each option can be used once, more than once or not at all. Only one option should be selected for each item.

Items:

1 A 75-year-old man who is a heavy smoker, with blood pressure of 170/105 mmHg, complains of floaters in the right eye for many months and flashing lights in bright sunlight. He has now noticed a 'curtain' across the vision in the right eye. ★ H

2 A 70-year-old woman complains of shadows which sometimes obscure her vision for a few minutes. She has felt unwell recently, with loss of weight and face pain when chewing food. ★ C

3 A 45-year-old woman, who is a heavy smoker with blood pressure of 170/110 mmHg, complains of impaired vision in the left eye. She has difficulty discriminating colours and has noticed that her eyes ache when looking to the side. ★ G

Current literature question

Current evidence concerning the effectiveness of routine mammography suggests that in the UK:

1 The screening age is lowered to 40
 false

2 Two-view mammography at each screening is cost-effective
 true

3 The screening interval is reduced to 2 years
 true

4 The mammograms should be read by two independent radiologists
 true

5 Mammography has been shown to be successful in reducing the mortality from breast cancer
 false

Apart from the subject preparation, it is important to practise answering MCQs and EMQs. All questions should be answered, particularly the true/false ones, where each candidate might get 50% right by random guessing alone. Time management is thus crucial. The candidate needs to be familiar with the definition of the common terms used in the paper given in Box 8.8, and to practise reading the question carefully, perhaps highlighting key words.

Consulting skills

This consists of an assessment of consulting skills based on video recordings. In exceptional circumstances, candidates unable to make a video tape (e.g. for religious or language reasons) may be examined in a simulated surgery of 'role-played' patients.

The video

The structure of the video assessment is designed to encourage good consulting and to complement training, rather than setting a minimum competence hurdle. The trainer and GP registrar reviewing consulting skills by watching and discussing video recordings is a well-established part of training. The only difference is that now the GP registrar is invited to present a tape showing what they can do for assessment in the MRCGP. Most of the preparation for the video will consist of trainer and GP registrar reflecting on and reviewing tapes, the GP registrar then trying out ideas for improvement and video recording the results—a process of continuing improvement.

When a candidate is satisfied with the performance, he or she presents the work in the form of a videotape of selected consultations, showing what they can do on a good day. The analogy is with an apprentice presenting a portfolio at the end of apprenticeship. The video is not an effective tool for looking at clinical skills, as patients may not attend with appropriately challenging problems. It is, however, good for assessing consultation skills, which tend to be consistent over a series of consultations. Not every consulting skill competency is relevant to every consultation, so the examiners look at a selection of consultations. The competencies are examined as outcomes rather than behaviours. This means there is no 'college' way of doing something. Many good doctors may achieve the same outcome by different approaches.

The candidate is required to present a video tape of 15 consultations, each of a maximum 15-minute length. Physical examinations of an intimate or sensitive nature should be held out of view of the camera. It is best to leave the camera running, as the continuing conversation may be relevant. The case mix should be selected to include at least two consultations with children under 10 years of age, and at least two consultations involving the management of chronic diseases in adults. The examiners are looking for the candidate's ability to demonstrate competencies, not trying to catch him or her out on mistakes. Serious errors would trigger discussion amongst the examiners. The competencies are least likely to appear in a tape of brief follow-up consultations and patients with sore throats. The selection should show a range of presentations and patients.

In addition to the tape, a workbook, supplied by the examination department, should be filled in, giving a log of the patients included. 'Consultation assessment forms' are supplied, on which the candidate adds relevant information, such as drugs prescribed, and has the opportunity to clarify details of the case that may not appear in the video clip. In five of the consultations, a more detailed evaluation of what went on in the consultation, minute by minute, is required.

Most trainers will wish to look at the final tape before it is presented. The examiners do not view this as cheating. An important aim of the video component is to improve consulting skills, so the more joint input from teacher and learner the better.

Table 8.3 details the competencies looked for by the examiners. The table describes five areas of competency and, within each, performance criteria (PC) which demonstrate aspects of each area of competence. The performance criteria are also labelled (P), for essential criteria involved in pass/fail decisions, and (M), desirable criteria required for the award of merit. The examiners look for evidence of these criteria in the tape, but do not expect them all to be present in all the consultations.

The simulated surgery

A small number of candidates may be unable to produce a video tape, for example for religious reasons. These candidates will be able to take a simulated surgery. This consists of a mock surgery with trained role-players as patients, each presenting a carefully

Table 8.3 Consulting skill competencies.

---

1. Discover the reasons for the patient's attendance

a. Elicit the patient's account of the (symptom(s) which made him/her turn to the doctor

(P) PC: *the doctor encourages the patient's contribution at appropriate points in the consultation*

(P) PC: *the doctor responds to clues*

b. Obtain relevant items of social and occupational circumstances

(P) PC: *the doctor elicits appropriate details to place the complaint(s) in a social and psychological context*

c. Explore the patient's health understanding

(M) PC: *the doctor takes the patient's health understanding into account*

d. Enquire about continuing problems

PC: *the doctor obtains enough information to assess whether a continuing complaint represents an issue which must be addressed in this consultation*

2. Define the clinical problem(s)

a. Obtain additional information about symptoms and details of medical history

(P) PC: *the doctor obtains sufficient information for no serious condition to be missed*

PC: *the doctor shows evidence of generating and testing hypotheses*

b. Assess the condition of the patient by appropriate physical or mental examination

(P) PC: *the doctor chooses an examination which is likely to confirm of disprove hypotheses which could reasonably have been formed **or** to address a patient's concern*

c. Make a working diagnosis

(P) PC: *the doctor appears to make a clinically appropriate working diagnosis*

3. Explain the problem(s) to the patient

a. Share the findings with the patient

(P) PC: *the doctor explains the diagnosis, management and effects of treatment*

b. Tailor the explanation to the patient

(P) PC: *the doctor explains in language appropriate to the patient*

(M) PC: *the doctor's explanation takes account of some or all of the patient's elicited beliefs*

c. Ensure that the explanation is understood and accepted by the patient

(M) PC: *the doctor seeks to confirm the patient's understanding*

Cont'd

Table 8.3 *(cont'd)*

---

4.   Address the patient's problem(s)

a.   Assess the severity of the presenting problem(s)

      PC: *the doctor differentiates between problems of differing degrees of severity and manages each appropriately*

b.   Choose an appropriate form of management

(P)   PC: *the doctor's management plan is appropriate for the working diagnosis, reflecting a good understanding of modern accepted medical practice*

c.   Involve the patient in the management plan to the appropriate extent

(P)   PC: *the doctor shares management options with the patient*

5.   Make effective use of the consultation

a.   Make efficient use of resources

      PC: *the doctor makes sensible use of available time and suggests further consultations as appropriate*

      PC: *the doctor makes appropriate use of other health professionals through investigations, referrals, etc.*

(P)   PC: *the doctor's prescribing behaviour is appropriate*

b.   Establish a relationship with the patient

(P)   PC: *the patient and doctor appear to have established a rapport*

c.   Give opportunistic health promotion advice

      PC: *the doctor deals appropriately with at-risk factors within the consultation*

From RCGP Assessment of Consulting Skills—Workbook and Instructions 1998.

thought out and tested patient scenario. The examiner observes and marks the consultation according to a marking schedule. The simulated surgery gives the opportunity to test clinical skills and examination skills in addition to consulting skills. Simple examinations may form part of the assessment, but more intimate examinations are not involved. Both role-players and candidates are fully briefed about how to conduct the surgeries. There is a break of a couple of minutes between each 10-minute case.

   The domains assessed in the simulated surgery include:

• Data gathering: the interview, history taking and physical examination.

• Communication: including explanation of symptoms and diagnosis, and agreeing the management.

- Management: appropriate and safe treatment and investigations.
- Anticipatory care: implications for patients and others, follow-up and safety-netting, health promotion and preventive care.

Simulated surgeries are also an excellent tool for formative assessment and teaching consulting and clinical skills. The organization and training of role-players involve a lot of preparation, and they are probably best organized within one or across several vocational training schemes.

The oral examination

This consists of two 20-minute orals and is a stand-alone module. The examiners will concentrate on professional decision-making skills in the context of patients, working in teams, the NHS and society as a whole, and on the values, attitudes and ethics that underlie practice.

There are two examiners at each oral examination, so the candidate will meet four examiners. There are typically five questions in each oral. All four examiners will have met earlier to plan the topic areas that each will cover. They will independently mark each candidate, but they also meet again after the orals, and in borderline situations they can review individual candidates' performance before agreeing the final score.

The examiners will aim to ask at least one question in each oral in each of the three main topic areas (see Box 8.9) and to spread their questions across the four contexts (see Box 8.10).

The examiners are looking for evidence that the candidate's approach to decision making is coherent, rational, ethical and sensitive.

There is often no single correct answer to a question. The good candidate will think aloud, showing the examiner how he or she develops the answer. It is often appropriate to give possible options before deciding on a final course of action. The examiners assess whether the candidate can see a range of possible solutions, assess the pros and cons of each, and then make a sensible decision, which need not necessarily be the one the examiner would have chosen.

The examiners are ultimately interested in how the candidate performs in real life, and may try to link theoretical concepts to

---

Box 8.9 Oral examination: topic areas

- Communication
- Professional values
- Personal and professional growth

Box 8.10 Oral examination: contexts

- Care of patients
- Working with colleagues and in teams
- General practice in society
- The doctor's personal responsibilities

---

the candidate's own practice. They are not impressed with a candidate who can quote all the references, but who has not thought critically about the information and fails to put it into practice.

Most questions will start with a short stem, and develop according to the examiners' planned topic area and the candidate's performance. The examiners' aim is to see how well a candidate can perform. It is often off-putting to be pushed hard for more, but this may mean things are going well and the examiners wish to see if the standard justifies a high mark.

The oral is a structured discussion between colleagues, and as such the candidate should incorporate the usual courtesies of such a dialogue. He or she should listen to the questions and ask for clarification if a question is not understood. Honesty counts. The examiners can soon spot the candidate who is making it up as he or she goes along, and sooner or later makes a statement that he or she regrets.

The examiners all work in the consulting room and know the realities of what can and cannot be done in the consultation, so be realistic.

The best preparation for the orals is to practise discussing relevant topics with colleagues and between trainer and GP registrar. Use the principles above to practise mock vivas.

The MRCGP is a well-researched, dynamic and continually evolving examination for good general practice. The only difference between preparing for a career in general practice and preparing to take the examination is gaining a familiarity with the structure of the examination.

Reference

Royal College of General Practitioners (1998) *Membership Examination Regulations*. RCGP, London.

Further reading

Clarke, R. & Croft, P. (1998) *Critical Reading for the Reflective Practitioner*. Butterworth-Heinemann, Oxford.

Moore, R. (1998) *MRCGP Examination*. RCGP, London.

Oxman, A.D., Sackett, D.L. & Guyatt, G.H. (1993) User's guide to the medical literature, I. How to get started. *Journal of the American Medical Association* **270**, 2598–2601.

Palmer, K.T. (1998) *Notes for the MRCGP*, 3rd edn. Blackwell Science, Oxford.

Ridsdale, L. (1995) *Evidence-based General Practice*. WB Saunders, Philadelphia.

Sackett, D.L., Haynes, R.B., Evyatt, G.H. & Tugwell, P. (1991) *Clinical Epidemiology—A Basic Science for Clinical Medicine*. Little, Brown, Boston.

Sackett, D.L., Richardson, W.S., Rosenberg, W. & Haynes, R.B. (1997) *Evidence-based Medicine—How to Practise and Teach EBM*. Churchill Livingstone, Edinburgh.

9 Evidence-based practice in primary care

Evidence-based health care: a definition at odds with its reputation?

You do not have to look far in the textbooks or on the Internet to find a definition of evidence-based health care (EBHC). One team of medical academics has defined it as 'the conscientious, judicious and explicit use of current best evidence in making decisions about the care of individual patients' (Sackett *et al.*, 1996). Another team has stated that 'evidence-based health care promotes the collection, interpretation, and integration of valid, important and applicable patient-reported, clinician-observed and research-derived evidence' (McMaster University internet site on evidence-based medicine http://www.hiru.mcmaster.c./ebm).

These quotes, and other accounts of what EBHC means to experts in the field, are often used as an entrée when teaching or learning about EBHC for the first time. But this worthy and rigorous starting-point fails to address the connotations that the term has for the non-expert. (Non-experts, remember, do not tend to read official definitions or explanations.)

Hannah-Rose Douglas interviewed a sample of GPs and practice nurses in 1997 and asked them what they thought of the expressions 'evidence-based medicine' and 'evidence-based health care'. She also interviewed people who regularly trained primary-care teams in EBHC and asked what kind of problems such individuals encountered on the training courses. The detailed methods and results of this qualitative study are reported elsewhere (Douglas & Greenhalgh, 1997), but, briefly, these findings, together with other studies conducted by ourselves and other researchers, suggest that EBHC has a number of associations for the non-academic primary-care practitioner.

To the primary-care practitioner, EBHC means some or all of the following:

- Attempting to keep up to date with as many clinical topics as possible.
- Attending (or, for many nurses, being sent on) academically demanding courses.
- Searching complex electronic databases for medical information (and becoming disillusioned when you do not find it).
- Becoming the victim of yet another dimension of central coercion and control.
- A long-winded way of demonstrating what is usually obvious to experienced clinicians.
- A counsel of perfection broadcast from ivory towers and with little regard for the practicalities of face-to-face consultations and long-term continuity of care.

I hope you can see that (with the exception of a growing body of enthusiasts) primary-care practitioners may not share the official perspective on EBHC. Many are suspicious and frightened of the 'evidence-based' approach to clinical practice. They may talk about it as an administrative rather than a professional task, which devalues rather than builds upon the experience gained after years in practice, and which entails an ever-receding goal of complete and comprehensive factual knowledge. They view it, in the words of one of our informants, as 'a big part of the problem rather than part or all of the solution'.

GPs and their staff have, over the past decade, experienced huge increases in out-of-hours workload, patient expectations, official paperwork (or the electronic equivalent) and demands from all sides for greater efficiency, effectiveness and accountability. The cry for them to become involved in EBHC tends to meet the same reaction as a cry for a more detailed income tax return or practice annual report.

This reaction is hardly surprising, but it reflects a fundamental misunderstanding of aspects of EBHC that are new and potentially useful. EBHC is **not** about knowing everything (or almost everything) or analysing every aspect of one's practice in order to become a perfect doctor. Indeed, one of the most balanced and entertaining articles on the philosophy of EBHC is subtitled 'feeling good about **not** knowing everything' (Slawson *et al.*, 1994).

Defining evidence-based health care: let's try again

EBHC is fundamentally about thinking logically and setting priorities. It is about distinguishing the **best** and **most relevant** evidence (which you need to read) from all the **other** evidence (which you can usually safely ignore).

Traditionally, we doctors played our hunches and based our management of the current patient more or less on what happened to the last patient with the same problem. The evidence-based approach encourages us to base our management on the accumulated results of hundreds or thousands of similar clinician–patient encounters—in other words, the research literature. When the focus of the analysis moves thus from individual case histories (anecdotes) to populations, the results allow us to express the possible outcomes of the different management options in the language of probability and risk (see Box 9.1).

Much of the published material on EBHC involves numbers and equations similar to those in Box 9.1, which you can practise for yourself. However, it would be quite wrong to dismiss the philosophy of EBHC as an exercise in mathematical reductionism by bright but inexperienced practitioners whose communication skills have mistakenly been honed on the Internet rather than at the bedside. To do so would be to miss the central contribution of the evidence-based healthcare movement to the quite remarkable revolution that is currently occurring in diagnostic, preventive and therapeutic care.

EBHC is not (or, at least, should not be) about subserving the patient's values and preferences to a rigid mathematical formula derived from some average effect on a distant population. However, it should be about **utilizing** mathematical formulae and other tools of clinical epidemiology to inform and refine the clinician's assessment of the pros and cons of different management options in the here and now. What is the diagnosis? Should I investigate? Should I treat? Should I refer? What would happen if I did nothing?

Thus, if I can presume to offer yet another definition of EBHC to the many that already exist in the literature, it would be:

Evidence-based health care is the enhancement of a
clinician's traditional skills in diagnosis, treatment,

prevention and related areas through the systematic framing of relevant and answerable questions and the use of mathematical estimates of probability and risk. Such estimates may be derived from an objective and complete appraisal of the relevant primary research literature, or from these same estimates presented as an overview, guideline, decision support system or other secondary source.

Box 9.1 Illustration of mathematical estimates of probability and risk derived from a randomized controlled trial of glyceryl trinitrate ointment in chronic anal fissure

The figures below are taken from a randomized controlled trial which compared the effect of glyceryl trinitrate vs. placebo ointment on healing rate in patients with chronic anal fissure (Lund & Scholefield, 1997). The equations are explained in more detail in Sackett *et al.* (1997).

	Healed at 8 weeks		
	Yes	No	Total
Control group	a = 3	b = 36	a + b = 39
Experimental group	c = 26	d = 12	c + d = 38

Control event rate (CER) = risk of outcome event in control group = a/(a + b) = 3/39 = 7.7%
Experimental event rate (EER) = risk of outcome event in experimental group = c/(c + d) = 26/38 = 68.4%
Absolute risk reduction (ARR) = CER − EER = 7.7% − 68.4% = −60.7%
Relative risk reduction (RRR) = (CER − EER)/CER = −60.7/7.7 = 78.9%
Number needed to treat (NNT) = 1/ARR = 1/(CER − EER) = 1/0.607 = **1.65**
i.e. Fewer than two people need to receive the drug in order for one person to achieve healing of the fissure—in other words, the treatment is highly effective

---

Box 9.2 The case of Mrs Griggs

Doctor: What can I do for you today?

Mrs Griggs: I think I've got an egg allergy.

Doctor: Mmmh. What makes you think that?

Mrs Griggs: I've brought an article to show you, doctor, from the evening paper. It says more and more people are getting allergic to eggs.

Doctor [quickly reading press cutting]: Do you have any symptoms?

Mrs Griggs: No. But it says here you can get a rash and all.

Doctor: Have you got a rash?

Mrs Griggs: No.

Doctor: Do eggs upset you in any way?

Mrs Griggs: Oh no, I love eggs. They've never upset me. That's why I came to ask you if it's OK to keep on having them.

Doctor: If eggs don't upset you, you can keep on having them, can't you?

Mrs Griggs: Thank you, doctor. That's all I wanted. Sorry to have troubled you.

Relevant evidence: how to spot it . . .

One major source of confusion among primary-care practitioners is what the term 'evidence' refers to. One perfectly legitimate form of evidence is the data you collect on your own patients when carrying out an audit (see Chapter 10)—for example, in response to the question 'How many of this practice's patients post myocardial infarction are taking regular low-dose aspirin?'. Indeed, in our own interviews, practice nurses almost invariably used the terms 'evidence' and 'research' to refer to data collected on their own patients rather than that produced in large clinical trials on someone else's patients (Douglas & Greenhalgh, 1997). Another perfectly valid use of the term evidence, discussed below and in Box 9.2, is patient-derived evidence about symptoms, concerns and expectations. Yet another form of evidence is the discussions you have with professional colleagues or the opinions expressed by experts.

However, in the language in which EBHC is generally presented by academic writers, the 'E' in EBHC refers to **published**

research evidence—that is, the finished product of a clinical trial or observational study. Published research evidence relevant to practising doctors usually falls into one of the following categories:

- Randomized controlled trials: most commonly trials that compare the effect of a drug treatment with that of placebo or a competitor.
- Cohort studies: subjects who have been exposed to a drug or toxin, such as a vaccine, tobacco or an environmental chemical, are followed up to see how many develop a particular disease or other outcome, compared with an unexposed cohort.
- Case-control studies: subjects who have developed a disease, as well as control subjects who have not, are asked about their exposure in the past to a putative causative agent.
- Case reports: a story about a particular event is told (most commonly these days, an adverse reaction to a drug).
- Surveys: something is measured in a group of patients (e.g. their blood pressure) or health professionals (e.g. their knowledge or attitudes).

Secondary research evidence, which is of particular interest to the busy GP, is material that sets out to summarize and draw conclusions from primary studies, for example:

- Journalistic (non-systematic) reviews: collect together some (but usually not all) primary evidence on a topic, usually interlaced with the author's personal opinion. Until very recently, most overviews were written by experts in the field and presented in this format, which has been described (A. Herxheimer, personal communication, 1998) as the tradition of 'eminence [sic] based health care'.
- Systematic reviews: **all** the evidence pertaining to a particular field of research is collected via a systematic search of the literature and unpublished sources, and evaluated using predefined quality criteria.
- Meta-analyses: systematic reviews in which the numerical results of different studies are combined using standard statistical techniques. Simply by increasing the numbers in the calculations, meta-analyses can make the estimate of the effect of an intervention both more precise (i.e. the possible limits of its magnitude are more tightly defined) and more definitive (i.e. we

can be much more confident that the result, whether positive or negative, is a true reflection of the effect studied rather than a result of chance).

- Guidelines: defined as systematically developed statements to assist practitioner decisions about appropriate health care for specific clinical circumstances (Field & Lohr, 1990).
- Economic analyses: studies involving the use of mathematical techniques to define choices in resource allocation.

A piece of secondary research is only as good as the primary studies which went into it and the techniques used for making sense of those studies, so the notion that anything that bears the title 'systematic review' or 'meta-analysis' **necessarily** counts as high-quality evidence is erroneous. Similarly, most GPs are all too aware that guidelines issued with the best intentions may or may not be valid or practicable. Current primary care guidelines for most conditions are based more on expert consensus than on primary research evidence. However, a number of major projects are under way, some organized through the Royal College of General Practitioners (RCGP), to develop genuinely evidence-based guidelines for primary care, so this situation is likely to change over the next decade.

This classification of the different forms of research is discussed in more detail elsewhere (Guyatt *et al.*, 1995; Greenhalgh, 1997).

. . . and where to find it

Anyone who qualified before about 1988 will have cut their researching teeth on the *Index Medicus*—a huge manual subject index that used to line the walls of medical libraries with its reddish-brown volumes. You could search the *Index Medicus* under the names of authors, or under particular topics (Medical Subject Headings), and probably under other key features as well. I last tried to look something up in the manual *Index Medicus* in about 1985, and I nearly dislocated my shoulder putting seven of its 18 volumes for that year back on the shelf. Fortunately, the whole database was made electronic soon afterwards and is now available on CD-ROM or directly over the Internet. The electronic version of the old *Index Medicus*, regularly updated by a team at the National Library of Medicine in the USA, is known as MEDLINE.

MEDLINE is accessed by a variety of commercial software packages; the most common are OVID, Silver Platter and Knowledge Finder. It is worth booking in for a half-day course in using this software at your local medical library (or attending the course run by the BMA Library in London). Some important sources of on-line evidence, in addition to MEDLINE, are listed in Table 9.1, along with some paper sources of secondary evidence.

The fourth column in Table 9.2 shows some suggested search strings for approaching the MEDLINE database using OVID software, based on the questions defined in the previous column. The details for searching MEDLINE are covered elsewhere (Greenhalgh, 1997), but you will see from the examples given here that there are a number of short cuts to the kind of rough-and-ready searching that we can achieve in day-to-day practice. For example:

- Use the textword search facility (type a key word such as 'hypertension' and add the suffix **.tw**) as well as (or instead of) MeSH terms to pick up any article containing that word in the title or abstract.
- Use subheadings as suggested by the software to limit the search to particular areas within a topic, such as 'diagnosis of', 'epidemiology of', etc.
- Combine two large searches using the Boolean operator 'and' (e.g. the search string ***epilepsy/and vigabatrin.tw** will give you articles indexed under 'epilepsy' as a subject heading and which contain the word 'vigabatrin'); use the 'limit set' options as suggested by the software to include or exclude particular study designs or publication types (e.g. you could limit the set to human subjects, English language, randomized trials, meta-analyses, and so on).

My own research suggests that only about a fifth of GPs are confident in using MEDLINE, and less than half have ever used it. However, finding research evidence is virtually impossible without the basic skills for accessing this important database. I predict that, within 5 years of the publication of this book, most GPs will have access to on-line sources of evidence (i.e. their desktop computer terminal will be connected to the Internet),

Table 9.1 Sources of research-based evidence for use in primary care.

Primary publications (journals which regularly publish randomized controlled trials and other robust research studies)
  British Medical Journal
  Lancet
  British Journal of General Practice
  Family Practice

Secondary publications (journals which summarize primary research in a format which allows rapid assimilation)
  Bandolier
  Effective Health Care Bulletins
  MeReC Bulletins
  Evidence-based Purchasing
  Evidence-based Medicine

Evidence-based health care on the Internet (web sites of electronic journals, search engines and academic departments of evidence-based practice with emphasis on primary care)
  British Medical Journal electronic edition: http://www.bmj.com

  Lancet electronic edition: http://www.thelancet.com

  Doctor's Desk (entry to Internet resources for EBHC presented in a GP-friendly way):
  http://drsdesk.sghms.ac.uk

  PubMed (free Medline service on the Internet):
  http://www4.ncbi.nlm.nih.gov/PubMed/clinical.html

  Biomednet search page: http://www.biomednet.com

  Sheffield Centre for Health and Related Research (SCHARR):
  http://www.shef.ac.uk/uni/academic/R-Z/sharr/ir/netting.html

  Unit for Evidence Based Practice and Policy (UCLMS/RFHSM):
  http://www.ucl.ac.uk/primcare-popsci/uebpp/uebpp.htm

---

so that time-consuming trips to the library will be a thing of the past. Elementary training in this area is probably the single most important way to spend a half-day's study leave if you are not already confident in the area.

Table 9.2 Formulating answerable questions and seeking evidence from consultations in primary care.

Example of patient problem seen in a GP consultation	Example of 'unfocused' question or reflection about the consultation	Example of focused question which might be answerable from research evidence	Suggested search string with which to approach MEDLINE database	Example of evidence (clinical trial, overview, guidelines, etc.)
Mother demands urgent visit after hours for child with earache 'so he can start the antibiotics tonight'	'I think I remember seeing a *BMJ* article on this subject recently'	In a well child with earache and clinical signs of acute otitis media, do the benefits of antibiotic treatment (in terms of symptom control and prevention of sequelae) outweigh the risks (expense and adverse effects)?	**otitis.tw** and **antibiotic.tw** and BMJ.jn and 97.yr (search by textwords, journal title and year for an article you know exists; combine sets using "and" operator)	Meta-analysis of RCTs of antibiotic vs placebo for acute otitis media (Del Mar *et al.*, 1997)
Taxi driver attends as emergency before surgery with facial droop identified as probable Bell's palsy	'I used to work for a consultant who gave high-dose steroids to people with this condition'	In a 53-year-old male with a presumed diagnosis of Bell's palsy, do the benefits (long-term cure) of high-dose oral steroid therapy outweigh the risks (adverse effects)?	***facial paralysis**/ or **Bell's Palsy.tw** and **random$.tw** (search by MeSH headings and textwords; merge sets using "or" operator)	Meta-analysis of RCTs of steroid versus placebo in Bell's palsy with commentary by a GP (Williamson & Whelan, 1996)

Clinical scenario	Reflection	Question	Search strategy	Evidence found
Elderly man with arthritis, recently bereaved, attends for no clear reason and leaves, dissatisfied. The doctor too feels dissatisfied with this consultation	'I guess he's depressed, but I wasn't sure how to handle it. It all seems so different in primary care compared with psychiatry outpatients'	In a 78-year-old male with a chronic painful condition and recent loss of spouse, what additional information should be sought to quantify the risk of significant depressive illness in the primary care situation?	***depression/di and primary care.tw** limit 1 to review articles (limit set by subheading 'diagnosis' and publication type 'review article')	Systematic overview of utility and ease of use of short questionnaires for case finding of depression in primary care (Mulrow et al., 1995)
'Drug rep' attends to offer information and prescribing incentives about a new antiepilepsy drug, vigabatrin	'He's clearly got a conflict of interest but he does sound convincing. How can I verify this sales pitch?'	In patients with a diagnosis of primary generalized epilepsy, what are the risks (costs, adverse effects) and benefits (fit control) of vigabatrin compared with current alternatives?	***epilepsy and random\$.tw and vigabatrin.tw** limit set to AIM journals (exclude industry-sponsored publications)	Systematic review of the effectiveness of new antiepileptic drugs (Marson et al., 1996)
Middle-aged teacher attends for results of blood tests sent on complaint of 'tired all the time'. All tests normal. Has leaflet from support group for myalgic encephalomyelitis	'What do I do now? She strikes me as a "familiar face, fat file" patient. I wonder if she'll ever get better?'	In a 38-year-old with no organic explanation for persistent tiredness, is there any association with psychiatric disorder and what is the prognosis for recovery?	***fatigue syndrome, chronic/ep and pt=review article** (map 'tiredness' to MeSH heading and limit set to epidemiology reviews)	Prospective cohort study of chronic fatigue symptoms in primary care (Wessely et al., 1996)

Tutorial exercise 1: Take five consecutive primary care consultations and prepare a table similar to that shown in Table 9.2. Focus particularly on converting your 'first impressions' of issues to consider into a three-part, answerable question about diagnosis, prognosis or therapy.

Clarifying your information needs

Professor David Sackett and colleagues have emphasized that EBHC involves, first of all, deciding what information you need to know (and don't) about a particular patient with a particular set of symptoms, beliefs, hopes and fears (Sackett *et al.*, 1997) (Fig. 9.1). Secondly, it requires you to seek appropriate information in a systematic and sensitive way. Note that, although the clinician's information needs in a particular case **may** be supplied in the form of factual, research-based journal articles accessed via the MEDLINE database, as shown in Table 9.2, there are times when the old-fashioned skills of empathic listening will provide crucial information about the presenting problem (and the patient's perspective on it). This is something that GPs, especially those with years of experience, are often very good at (see Box 9.2).

A less experienced doctor, when faced with Mrs Griggs's initial query in Box 9.2, might see this problem in terms of the 'evidence' for the food allergy hypothesis presented in the newspaper article. But the GP in the story uses his traditional consulting skills to explore the preliminary question 'what do I need to know (and don't)....', and finds that the main information gap is the patient's reason for attending. In the systematic search for the relevant information, he helps the patient define her problem more precisely, and thereby solve it herself. Although this consultation is not, on the face of it, 'evidence-based', it clearly illustrates how a logical approach can obviate, rather than generate, a sophisticated search for research evidence.

Of course, a newly defined patient problem very often does produce a need for published research evidence. Table 9.2 gives five examples of problems commonly seen in primary-care consultations. Also, examples of unfocused ('first-impression') questions that a new practitioner may ask, more focused questions with which he or she might approach sources of evidence, and

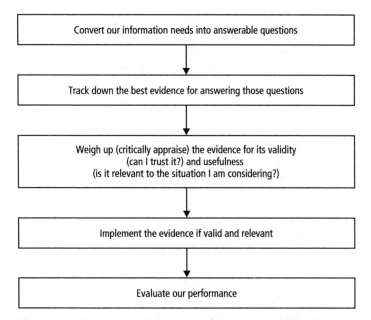

Figure 9.1 The recommended sequence for practising evidence-based health care (see Sackett *et al.*, 1991).

some references for high-quality evidence that could be found from appropriate sources are provided. In my experience, too little emphasis is often given in EBHC training to the proper framing of an answerable question—on how to convert the hunches and reflections listed in the second column in Table 9.2 to the focused and answerable questions in the third column.

Framing questions such as these may be easier if you divide them into three parts, as described by Sackett *et al.* (1991). First, define the patient or patient population ('How would I describe a person similar to this one?'). Next, define what will happen to this group ('By what manoeuvre or event will the study group be characterized?'—e.g. taking a particular drug), and, if relevant, what manoeuvre or event will characterize the comparison or control group. Finally, define a particular (hopefully, patient-relevant) outcome you believe might be influenced by this manoeuvre.

Thus, when patients ask us a question about a drug treatment, such as 'Will these tablets make me better?', we must rephrase the question to read something like: 'In a white male patient aged

64 with Type 2 diabetes but no other coexisting condition, will a course of famciclovir at recommended dosage alleviate the symptoms of shingles and prevent postherpetic neuralgia?'. Similarly, the question 'is it okay for Jimmy to have his jab?', should be expressed as: 'In a healthy 3-month-old infant with a normal birth history and mild atopic eczema but no other illness, what is the long-term risk of serious adverse events following routine triple (diphtheria, tetanus and pertussis) vaccination?'.

Evidence and uncertainty in primary care

You may well discover, when you try the exercise above, that your list contains problems that cannot be classified. The realities of primary care are such that it often seems impossible to define a single answerable question that will act as the key to a particular diagnostic puzzle. Kieran Sweeney has reviewed a number of studies which suggest that between a third and a half of all GP consultations concern 'non-diagnoses' and 'non-diseases'—ill-defined and generally self-limiting symptoms which bear little or no relation to the discrete disease entities described in medical textbooks (Sweeney, 1996).

Marshall Marinker observed a fundamental difference between the practice of medicine in primary as opposed to secondary care, which arises, of course, from the much higher prevalence of organic disease in secondary care. The diagnostic task of the specialist, says Marinker, is to reduce uncertainty, to explore possibility and to marginalize error. In contrast, the task of the GP, is to accept uncertainty, to explore probability and to marginalize danger (discussed by Marinker in the 1994 Bayliss Lecture, 'The end of general practice', given to the RCGP in 1994). In other words, specialists tend to perform investigations in order to confirm their suspicion of organic disease, while GPs usually perform investigations in order to confirm their suspicion of the **absence** of organic disease, and hence to reassure.

This argument has been used to support the claim that EBHC is less relevant in the 'softer' branches of medicine than in the specialties (Bradley & Field, 1995; Schon, 1995; Sweeney, 1996). My own view is that the reverse is true. It is precisely **because** we deal for the most part with non-diagnoses and non-diseases that we GPs must make assiduous use of both logic and the tools of clinical epidemiology. But, because the signal-to-noise ratio is so much lower in primary care, we should not expect this task to be easy.

As you can see from the last two examples in Table 9.2, not only is it possible to formulate answerable questions about non-diseases, but it is also possible to address those questions through well-designed research studies based in primary care. Given that an increasing proportion of research funding is now being directed at primary care, the evidence base which GPs will be able to draw upon in the future is set to increase substantially.

Critical appraisal skills—necessary but not sufficient for evidence-based practice

The process of digesting and interpreting the information from published sources has become known (especially amongst MRCGP examiners) by the turgid expression 'critical appraisal'. This simply means 'using your common sense and a checklist of questions to decide if a medical journal article is both valid (can you trust it?) and relevant (does it apply to the patient, or patient population, you are considering right now?)'. There are many books and journal articles on critical appraisal (Greenhalgh, 1997; Sackett *et al.*, 1997), and an increasing number of workshops and distance-learning courses which introduce you to the finer points of the subject. Box 9.3 reproduces a checklist which could be used for assessing the methods section of a clinical trial.

It is important to recognize, however, that, although critical appraisal skills are frequently equated with EBHC in the run-up to MRCGP, evidence-based practice is much more than the ability to pick holes in published research papers. It is, many would argue, a way of thinking—an approach to systematically defining and addressing your own information needs and utilizing that information appropriately and consistently in patient care.

Many practitioners would argue that the really difficult part of EBHC is concerned with implementation. This difficulty can be either in the individual consultation (what treatment did I offer Mr Smith for his non-ulcer dyspepsia, and what were the practical barriers to treating him according to the best evidence?) or in the practice policy (having looked up the evidence to make a decision about Mr Smith, what general policy should we adopt in our practice for treating non-ulcer dyspepsia in other patients?).

Box 9.3 Checklist for evaluating the methods section of
a published paper

1 Was the study original?
2 Who is the study about?
   • how were subjects recruited?
   • who was included in, and who was excluded from, the study?
   • were the subjects studied in 'real life' circumstances?
3 Was the design of the study sensible?
   • what intervention or other manoeuvre was being considered?
   • what outcome(s) were measured, and how?
4 Was the study adequately controlled?
   • if a 'randomized trial', was randomization truly random?
   • if a cohort, case-control or other non-randomized comparat-
     ive study, were the controls appropriate?
   • were the groups comparable in all important aspects except for
     the variable being studied?
   • was assessment of outcome (or, in a case-control study, alloca-
     tion of casemix) 'blind'?
5 Was the study large enough, and continued for long enough, and
was follow-up complete enough, to make the results credible?

(Reproduced from Greenhalgh (1997) with permission of the
publisher)

Tutorial exercise 2: Using the checklist in Box 9.3, decide whether
a particular paper you have chosen from the literature is valid and
relevant to a practical decision you have to make about a patient
problem.

The detailed analysis of how to implement change in professional practice and how to influence policy making for clinical effectiveness is beyond the scope of this chapter and is
covered elsewhere (Laffel & Blumenthal, 1989; Haines & Donald,
1998; Appleby *et al.,* 1995; Oxman *et al.*, 1995; Greenhalgh, 1997).
A number of important principles, however, should be noted
(Appleby *et al.*, 1995):
• Prerequisites for implementing changes for EBHC in clinical
  practice are nationally available research evidence and clear,
  robust and local justification for change.

- All interested parties should be consulted and involved, and led by a respected product champion.
- The knock-on effects of change in one sector (e.g. acute services) to others (e.g. general practice or community care) should be addressed.
- Contracts (e.g. between purchasers and providers) are best used to summarize agreement that has already been negotiated elsewhere, not to table points for discussion.
- Implementing evidence may save neither time nor money.

Conclusion: is my practice evidence-based?

Evidence-based health care, especially as defined on pages 145 and 146, is not a passing fad. It should not be viewed as a threat either to patient choice or to the traditional objectives and values of the family doctor service. Box 9.4 gives a context-sensitive

---

Box 9.4 Is my practice evidence-based? A context-sensitive checklist for individual clinical encounters

1 Have I identified and prioritized the clinical, psychological, social and other problem(s), taking into account the patient's perspective?
2 Have I performed a sufficiently competent and complete examination to establish the likelihood of competing diagnoses?
3 Have I considered additional problems and risk factors which may need opportunistic attention?
4 Have I, where necessary, sought evidence (from systematic reviews, guidelines, clinical trials and other sources) pertaining to the problems?
5 Have I assessed and taken into account the completeness, quality and strength of the evidence?
6 Have I applied valid and relevant evidence to this particular set of problems in a way that is both scientifically justified and intuitively sensible?
7 Have I presented the pros and cons of different options to the patient in a way he or she can understand, and incorporated the patient's utilities into the final recommendation?
8 Have I arranged review, recall, referral or other further care as necessary?

(Reproduced from Greenhalgh (1997) with permission of the publisher)

---

checklist that should allow professional experience and intuition to be integrated with the appropriate use of research evidence in the primary-care consultation.

References

Appleby, J., Walshe, K. & Ham, C. (1995) *Acting on the Evidence: A Review of Clinical Effectiveness: Sources of Information, Dissemination and Implementation.* NAHAT, Birmingham.

Bradley, F. & Field, J. (1995) Evidence based medicine [letter]. *Lancet* **346**, 838–839.

Del Mar, C., Glasziou, P. & Hayem, M. (1997) Are antibiotics indicated as initial treatment for children with acute otitis media? A metaanalysis. *British Medical Journal* **314**, 1526–1529.

Douglas, H.-R. & Greenhalgh, T. (1997) *Life's Too Short and the Evidence Too Hard to Find: a Training Needs Analysis of GPs and Practice Nurses in Evidence-Based Health Care.* North Thames Regional Office, London.

Field, M.J. & Lohr, K.N. (1990) *Clinical Practice Guidelines: Direction of a New Agency.* Institute of Medicine, Washington, DC.

Greenhalgh, T. (1997) *How to Read a Paper: The Basics of Evidence-based Health Care.* BMJ Publishing Group, London.

Guyatt, G.H., Sackett, D.L., Sinclair, J.C., Hayward, R., Cook, D.J. & Cook, R.J. (1995) Users' guides to the medical literature. IX. A method for grading health care recommendations. *Journal of the American Medical Association* **274**, 1800–1804.

Haines, A. & Donald, A. (eds) (1998) *Getting Research Findings into Practice.* BMJ Publishing Group, London.

Laffel, G. & Blumenthal, D. (1989) The case for using industrial quality management science in health care organizations. *Journal of the American Medical Association* **262**, 2869–2873.

Lund, J.N. & Scholefield, J.H. (1997) A randomised, double-blind, placebo-controlled trial of glyceryl trinitrate ointment in treatment of anal fissure. *Lancet* **349**, 11–14.

Marson, A.G., Kadir, Z.A. & Chadwick, D.W. (1996) New anti-epileptic drugs: a systematic review of their efficacy and tolerability. *British Medical Journal* **313**, 1169–1174.

Mulrow, C.D., Williams, J.W., Jr, Gerety, M.B., Ramirez, G., Montiel, O.M. & Kerber, C. (1995) Case-finding instruments for depression in primary care settings. *Annals of Internal Medicine* **122**, 913–921.

Oxman, A., Davis, D., Haynes, R.B. & Thomson, M.A. (1995) No magic bullets: a systematic review of 102 trials of interventions to help health professionals deliver services more effectively or efficiently. *Canadian Medicine Association Journal* **153**, 1423–1443.

Sackett, D.L., Haynes, R.B., Guyatt, G.H. & Tugwell, P. (1991) *Clinical Epidemiology—A Basic Science for Clinical Medicine*, 2nd edn. Little, Brown, London.

Sackett, D.L., Rosenberg, W.M.C., Gray, J.A.M., Haynes, R.B. & Richardson, W.S. (1996) Evidence-based medicine: what it is and what it isn't. *British Medical Journal* **312**, 71–72.

Sackett, D.L., Richardson, W.S., Rosenberg, W. & Haynes, R.B. (1997) *Evidence Based Medicine: How to Practice and Teach EBM*. Churchill Livingstone, London.

Schon, D.A. (1995) *The Reflective Practitioner—How Professionals Think in Action*, 3rd edn. Basic Books, Kings Lynn.

Slawson, D.C., Shaughnessy, A.F. & Bennett, J.H. (1994) Becoming a medical information master: feeling good about not knowing everything. *Journal of Family Practice* **5**, 505–513.

Sweeney, K. (1996) Evidence and uncertainty. In: *Sense and Sensibility* (ed M. Marinker). BMJ Publishing Group, London.

Wessely, S., Chalder, T., Hirsch, S., Wallace, P. & Wright, D. (1996) Psychological symptoms, somatic symptoms, and psychiatric disorder in chronic fatigue and chronic fatigue syndrome: a prospective study in the primary care setting. *American Journal of Psychiatry* **153**, 1050–1059.

Williamson, I.G. & Whelan, T.R. (1996) The clinical problem of Bell's palsy: is treatment with steroids effective? *British Journal of General Practice* **46**, 743–747.

10 Audits, projects and research

Introduction

Mere utterance of the words 'research and audit' often leads to the cry: 'It's not real general practice—it's too academic!' In reality, both research and audit are inextricably linked with providing patient care and the principles are relevant to all practising GPs. Think back to a typical surgery. The first patient is a 26-year-old woman with symptoms of cystitis; you wonder whether an MSU should be taken and what the chances are that there may be an abnormality. The next patient is a 68-year-old man whom you find to have a raised blood pressure (BP) of 210/115. There appears to be no record of a previous BP measurement, although he has had several consultations before. You wonder whether this lack of BP recording is typical of your practice.

The young woman presents a research question—'What is the right thing to do?'; and the older man presents an audit question—'Is the right thing being done?'. Both research and audit depend on having a spirit of enquiry and require appropriate methods of measurement and data collection, but there are differences (see Table 10.1).

Table 10.1

Research	Audit
Discovers the right thing to do	Determines whether the right thing is being done
A series of 'one-off' projects	A cyclical series of reviews
Collects complex data	Collects routine data
Experiment rigorously defined	Review of what clinicians actually do
Often possible to generalize from findings	Not possible to generalize from findings

What is the value of research and audit projects?

A substantial degree of commitment and time is necessary to ensure successful completion of research and audit projects—so why bother?

- An audit project is required for the purposes of summative assessment. This is usually the compelling reason.
- Both projects lead to improved quality of patient care, not just as an outcome but by the very process of carrying out the project.
- The process acts as an aid to continuing medical education, identifying learning needs and developing increased awareness.
- There is a sense of personal and professional achievement, which may lead to publication, and the opportunity to put something different on your CV.

What is audit?

The aim of audit is to improve clinical care through a systematic critical analysis of the procedures used for the diagnosis and treatment, the use of resources and the resulting outcome and quality of life of the patient. There are various definitions, but in all descriptions of audit a basic method can be identified—the audit cycle (see Fig. 10.1). Three basic steps can be identified:

1 What should be happening? In the first place some kind of statement is made about what should be happening, developing criteria and standards.

2 What is happening? The next step is to perform an investigation to find out exactly what is happening, as opposed to what we would like to think is happening.

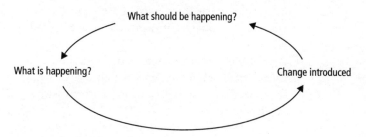

Figure 10.1 The audit cycle.

3 Introducing change. The **real** value of audit is the introduction of whatever changes are necessary in order to make sure that what is happening does comply with what is expected. Once this phase has been implemented the cycle is repeated, some would say indefinitely!

The educational benefit from audit

There are several educational strengths of audit. First, a critical review of current practice and the setting of standards encourages updating of a wide variety of areas. Second, audit highlights the need for specific knowledge/information, the acquisition of new skills and the development of existing ones, and the need to undertake research. Third, participation in small working groups is effective in modifying attitudes and, fourth, self-evaluation (the judgement of one's own performance) is made possible through audit and is at the heart of continuing professional development.

Audit is able to promote learning by asking the participant four simple questions:

1 What am I doing?
2 How am I doing it?
3 Why am I doing it in that way?
4 Can I do it better or differently?

How to carry out an audit

For an audit to be successful and worth the valuable time and effort spent on it, certain basic principles need to be considered:

- **A worker-centred approach.** The central feature is the adoption of a 'no-blame' approach, associated with a joint responsibility for the choice and planning of the audit. This ensures commitment and a greater chance of producing change if required.
- **A problem-solving approach.** Audit should concentrate on issues that are important and that need to be sorted out, rather than spending a lot of time concentrating on projects that have no clear purpose.

As a rule audit does not need ethical committee approval, because the treatment given is that which would be normally given for the benefit of the individual patient.

An audit is divided into a number of distinct stages to ensure a systematic approach. This prevents subsequent mistakes that can be costly in time and resources.

Stage 1: Identifying the problem

This is probably the most important stage, especially if the outcome of the audit is to have any real and lasting benefit for patient care. The problem should be important, likely to benefit patients and the practice, have potential for improvement and be worth the effort in both the time and the resources required to complete it!

Problems often arise out of everyday practice—a patient makes a complaint, an error is noted or there is a feeling that things could, and should, have been done better. The scope and potential for audit can be best appreciated by considering:

- **Structure.** This refers to the inputs to care, including manpower, premises and facilities. Examples include the availability and accessibility of doctors and practice nurses. 'Are the number of emergency appointments sufficient to cope with demand?'
- **Process.** This refers to the activities of providing care, looking at what is done and how it is done. Examples include appropriateness to the patient or compliance. 'Do all insulin-dependent diabetic patients know how to deal with hypoglycaemia?'
- **Outcome.** This refers to the result of the clinical intervention. Examples include improved health indicators and quality of life for patients. 'Are we achieving immunization targets for the under-5s?'

Depending on the chosen area that is to be considered, appropriate methods for observing care are required. These may be direct, for example video recording consultations or sitting in reception, or indirect, for example reviewing records, reports from patients and patient-satisfaction surveys.

Stage 2: Setting priorities

The highest priorities are those that significantly improve patient care. One priority is situations that put patients' lives at risk: for example, requests for emergency home visits.

Stage 3: Choosing a method

A method of collecting information has to be considered. What needs to be collected, how it needs to be collected and in what form, for example electronic or manual, and, probably most importantly, who is going to collect it! It is vital to keep the method simple and only collect information that is absolutely essential; otherwise valuable time will be wasted and you will end up with so much data that you cannot make sense out of them! At this stage, it is important to be clear about what information you will be collecting and how much you will be delegating (or dumping!) on to others.

Stage 4: Setting criteria and standards

This stage is when you can say what should be happening. A **criterion** is an item of care or some aspect of the practice that can be used to assess quality. The criterion should be expressed in a statement, for example 'all adult patients with epilepsy should be seen yearly'. To make this statement useful for the purpose of improving care it needs some clarification, and we need to define a **standard**, which is a statement of the proportion of occasions or patients that need to fulfil this criterion. For example, for the above criterion we may state 'that 80% of adults with epilepsy must be seen yearly'.

How to decide on the appropriate criteria and standards is obviously problematical. Ideally this should be the minimum acceptable standard—the level which you would be ashamed to fall below in the care of an ordinary patient. After all, it is possible to raise the standard for subsequent audits! The setting of criteria and standards may be predetermined: for example, cervical cytology or immunization rates. Alternatively, criteria and standards may have to be developed by discussion with the practice team and colleagues, by taking into account what literature or protocols state (e.g. the British Thoracic Society guidelines for asthma), and considering how they can be reasonably applied to your practice and its patient population. There is nothing more demoralizing than not being able to reach impossibly high standards through no fault of your own.

It is easier to make one or two important statements than to have a whole range that cannot be worked through. There is always the opportunity to return to the topic.

Stage 5: Comparing actual performance with criteria and standards to determine deficiencies

At this point, the information collected in stage 3 is used to identify any areas of care which are below the predetermined standard—this can be called a deficiency in care. The collected information needs to be analysed and presented and this is discussed later in this chapter.

Stage 6: Designing and implementing actions to remedy identified deficiencies

The results are presented, compared with the standard and an action plan designed to overcome the deficiencies in care. It has to be decided what needs to be done, how it needs to be done, who is going to do it and when it is going to be done.

Stage 7: Re-evaluating care to ensure that remedial action has been effective

Failure to complete the audit cycle is the usual reason for audit failing to improve care, and the majority of audits that are done or presented in practice reports or publications have not been around the full audit cycle (see Fig. 10.2). Obviously this part of the cycle takes time to complete and it is not usually expected to be carried out in the audit project for summative assessment purposes.

Sources of help when carrying out an audit project

Your trainer should be able to give you all the advice you require, combined with some background reading. Each district will have a medical audit advisory group (MAAG), which is a multidisciplinary group that has particular interest and expertise in medical audit.

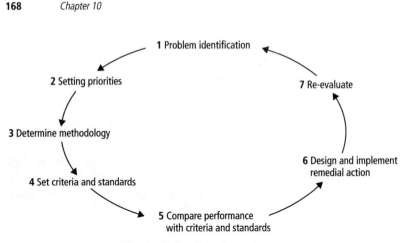

Figure 10.2 The detailed audit cycle.

Carrying out your summative assessment audit project

The choice of audit should, where possible, be chosen with the guidance of your trainer and based on the advice given above. The current audit should not have been performed before in that practice and the trainer will be responsible for authenticating the originality of your work. However, you can call upon reasonable help, for example in the data collection or if you need technical advice, for example with statistics. It is anticipated that you will begin to form ideas about the area you would like to audit within the first 2 months of your general practice attachment. This will mean learning the theoretical aspects of how to do an audit early in the training year, either from the day-release course or from your trainer.

Once you have decided on an audit question, you need to plan the method, standard setting and data collection. Data collection should probably take no more than 2 weeks. The next 6 weeks should be devoted to writing up the audit and submission. In other words, the whole project should be able to be completed in the first 6 months of your general practice attachment. This short timescale will necessarily determine the complexity of the audit that you can reasonably undertake in your training year, bearing in mind the other competing demands on your time. It is usually impossible to complete the whole of the audit cycle, given these factors, but you will be expected to have discussed the implementation of change and re-evaluation stages in your report.

Writing up your summative assessment audit project

The submission should be typed and written in concise English and should normally be between 1500 and 3000 words. Figures and graphs may be used to support results and conclusions. The author of the submission should be clearly identifiable and there should be a statement that the work is that only of this named doctor. The work needs to have each page numbered and presented in order and suitably bound together.

Title

The title should give an indication of the area of clinical activity audited and the audit question: for example, 'The surveillance of adults with asthma: do we conform to the British Thoracic Society's Guidelines?'.

Summary

The summary should be written under the following headings:
- The aim of the audit.
- The criteria and standards to be used.
- The method used.
- The results obtained.
- The main conclusions and implications for future practice.

Introduction

The introduction should include:
- A statement about how this area of audit came to be important to you and to the practice, for example following a patient complaint. This should be followed by a review of the relevant background literature with references to the major studies and reports in this area. A literature search at the local medical library or the RCGP library may be necessary.
- The aim of the audit and the audit question, which should be clearly stated.

Criteria and standards

The criteria to be measured should be stated with reference to why you chose them. The standards against which your criteria are being judged should be stated and reasons given for your choice, for example suggested by royal colleges, discussion in practice or local guidelines.

Method of data collection and analysis

The method of data collection and analysis should be clearly stated. If sampling methods were used, it should be stated how this was done, including a justification of the approach. The method of analysis should be clearly stated.

Results

The results should contain a presentation of all the relevant results and tabulation and any statistical tests should be used appropriately. There should be a detailed explanation of how any data were analysed.

Discussion

The discussion should include the following:
- The choice of criteria and standards, their advantages, limitations and alternatives.
- The method used, including the advantages and limitations of that method, for example the validity and reliability of the measurements and the possible sources of bias. Possible alternative methods can be discussed.
- The results and a reflection on the difficulties in interpreting those results, for example the response to questionnaires.
- The reasons why the measured performance has fallen short of the original standard.
- The appropriate conclusions and implications for the practice in terms of suggested areas where changes are needed. If no changes are suggested, this opinion should be justified in the light of the stated reasons for undertaking the audit in the first place.

- A clear plan of change and a strategy for implementation. The potential problems and obstacles should be identified and strategies described for overcoming them. If performance has been satisfactory, you should discuss the factors in the practice that facilitated this.
- A clear statement of how the author intends to review the changes to assess whether the performance has been improved. If no changes are suggested, then you should speculate on which audit questions should be approached next.

References

References should be up to date and able to be traced by others. They should be in either Vancouver or Harvard style:
- Vancouver style: numbered in the order in which they appear in the text and arranged in numerical order in the reference list.
- Harvard style: references in the text shown as '(author(s) and date of publication)' and arranged in alphabetical order in the reference list.

Table 10.2 provides a guideline of the schedule used for marking the summative assessment audit project.

What is research?

Research covers all activities involved in the planned, systematic collection and/or analysis of data to answer a specific question or test a precise hypothesis. Increasingly we are all expected to base our professional practice—what we do day to day—on research evidence. Sometimes research is available and well validated and we can use it to inform decision making, but at other times the only answer may be to find out for yourself.

In health-care research the primary intention is to advance knowledge to enable patients, in general, to benefit. The individual patient may or may not benefit directly. Any research involving patients directly needs ethical committee approval, and a research protocol must be submitted to the local research ethics committee for approval before the research project begins. The local research ethics committee can be contacted through the Local Medical Committee (LMC) or the postgraduate centre.

Table 10.2 Summative assessment audit project marking schedule.

Question	Criterion

Why was the audit done?	Reason for choice
	    Should be clearly defined and reflected in the title
	    Should include potential for change

How was the audit done?	Criteria chosen
	    Should be relevant to the subject of the audit
	    Should be justified, e.g. literature
	Preparation and planning
	    Should show appropriate teamwork and methodology in carrying out the audit
	If standards are set they should be appropriate and justified

What was found?	Interpretation of data Should use all relevant data to allow appropriate conclusions to be drawn
What next?	Detailed proposals for change Should show explicit details of proposed changes

How to carry out a research project

The first question to ask yourself before embarking on a research project is 'Why am I doing this in the first place? Do I have the time and the commitment to see the project through, especially given all the other conflicting demands on my time?'

Once you are clear in your mind what you may be letting yourself in for, you need to consider certain questions.

What is the purpose of the study?
What are the aims and the precise objectives? What question do you want to be answered? Is the purpose to evaluate an intervention, for example treatment, service or procedure? Or is the purpose to investigate a possible association between various factors, for example smoking and home visits for childhood coughs and colds?

What is known about the problem?
What are the gaps in our present knowledge? How will the study contribute to a new understanding of the problem?

Are you going to carry out a pilot project first?
This is really essential before you embark on a study, as it avoids costly mistakes both financially and in time wasted. Often difficulties cannot be adequately predicted and subsequent alterations to the main study can spell overall success or failure. Usually some form of pilot is essential if you wish to obtain any form of substantial funding.

What design will be used in the project?
Will the study be a survey or observational study or will it be a 'trial' (or 'intervention') of a treatment, procedure or service. Will it be a case–control study, cross-sectional study or cohort study, or will it be an intervention study, for example randomized controlled trial?

The chosen method will be determined by the focus of the research question, and requires further reading or expert advice.

How are the subjects of the study to be chosen?
What is the population from which the subjects will be drawn, for example all middle-class bankers or young New Age travellers? Is it all this population or is a sample to be taken? If so, how is this sample to be taken and will this sample be representative of the study population? What is the method of obtaining a random sample?

Attention needs to be paid particularly to the selection criteria, the sampling methods and the number of subjects needed to obtain a significant result.

What data need to be collected, and why?
What factors (variables) are thought to affect the outcome? Are there any factors that could distort the outcome? For example, a study looking at the uptake of a practice-run contraception clinic may be seriously distorted if a major national health education campaign is in progress. What are the measures of outcome of the trial and are they clear and unambiguous? For example, what is

meant by the term 'stroke'—is it a cerebral haemorrhage, infarction, embolism, transient ischaemic attack or bleed into a brain tumour?

The amount of data collected should be restricted to that which is required to answer the research question; otherwise you can end up with large amounts of data that cannot be analysed and from which no clear conclusions can be drawn.

What is the 'intervention' in the study and how are the variables to be defined and measured?
The intervention in intervention studies should be clearly defined and consistently applied to the whole of the chosen study group, regardless of whether it is a treatment or service. The variables, such as social class, ethnic origin and age, should be clearly defined and reflect those used in comparable studies or, if not, the reasons for the differences should be stated.

How are the data to be collected and measurements to be made?
This is discussed later in this chapter.

How will the data be analysed and presented?
This is discussed later in this chapter.

What are the ethical considerations?
Are the rights of patients properly observed and respected? Do I have the approval of the local research ethics committee?

The project plan

Finally, you need to develop a project plan. The plan should consider the estimated time required for each of the stages and the project as a whole, and the resource implications (not only the likely financial costs, but also the time and resources provided by yourself and any others involved in the study). It should also give a clear impression of any expert help that you will need.

Sources of help and funding for your research project

Your first port of call should be your trainer, but additional help can be obtained from local academic departments of general practice and the RCGP, either centrally or locally in the faculty.

Writing up your research project

There is a recognized format for writing up your research, but if you are planning to submit it for publication you will usually find that a particular style is required. These details can be obtained from the relevant publication who will normally provide 'Instructions to authors' guidance. The usual format is as follows:

• Introduction.
• Methods.
• Results.
• Analysis.
• Discussion and conclusion.

For guidance on the content of each section look at any respectable relevant publication.

Collection, analysis and presentation of data for audit and research

Both audit and research involve measuring or recording certain characteristics, which are under observation and from which it is hoped to be able to draw certain conclusions. The information collected is usually in the form of **quantitative** data, in which the data are numerical and can be analysed by various statistical tests. Some examples are: (i) simple counts of the number of patients who improved or did not improve after a certain intervention; (ii) the number of patients who reported satisfaction or dissatisfaction following the introduction of a particular service; or (iii) the number of patients who were not seen each year when a standard had been set that they should be seen. Such data are limited because certain outcomes, such as a patient's subjective experiences, cannot be represented. **Qualitative** data refer to narrative descriptions of events, such as the experiences of mothers attending antenatal classes, and are analysed by looking for underlying themes; it is not possible to apply statistical tests, but numerical data can be useful in supplying supportive evidence. It is recommended that, if qualitative research methods are being contemplated, the investigator obtains appropriate expert advice to ensure validity (that is, do they actually measure what is intended) and reliability (that is, can they be repeated to yield the same results).

Analysis may be simple, in the form of descriptive statistics, for example total numbers or average and percentage. This can be easily presented in the form of tables, pie charts and bar charts. The purpose of clear presentation is to highlight key points and to assist in the accurate interpretation of data and this is especially important if the presentation is being shown to others.

Interpretative statistics are required when it is necessary to draw inferences about the population from which a sample has been taken or when it is not readily apparent that the result is actually significantly different from what would occur by chance. Appropriate statistical tests need to be employed in such circumstances, but these are beyond the scope of this chapter and specialist books should be consulted.

Conclusion

Success in carrying out and completing an audit or research project depends on **your** enthusiasm and commitment. It is a valuable and powerful learning opportunity, but equally it is important not to underestimate the hurdles along the way.

Remember:
- Getting started will take twice as long as the data collection.
- Completion of the project usually takes twice as long as you originally estimated.
- A level of tedium will develop, which seems to increase as the project progresses.
- No project ever runs smoothly.
- At the end of the project you will always have regrets and wish that you had done it differently.

Despite all of this people do get hooked on research and audit, and this begs the question—Why?

There appears to be a natural curiosity about what we do in our day-to-day work: 'Why is that so?', 'What would happen if I did such and such?', 'Are my experiences similar to or different from those of other doctors?' and 'Can I improve the care of my patients?' Audit and research are an integral part of good medical practice and are not a sterile activity divorced from clinical work and only performed by people wearing anoraks bent over their computers!

Further reading

Armstrong, D. & Grace, J. (1995) *Research Methods and Audit in General Practice*. Oxford University Press, Oxford.

Beaglehole, R., Bonita, R. & Kjellstrom, T. (1993) *Basic Epidemiology*. WHO, Geneva.

Edwards, A. & Talbot, R. (1994) *The Hard-Pressed Researcher*. Addison Wesley Longman, London.

Irvine, D. & Irvine, S. (1997) *Making Sense of Audit*, 2nd Edn. Radcliffe Medical Press, Oxford.

11 The practice as a small business within the NHS

One of the experiences which new registrars least expect on commencement of their trainee year is the introduction to the world of the small business. Nothing in their previous experience or formal education will have prepared them for practice meetings in which the main item on the agenda is the cost of a new electric barrier to the surgery car park or the malfunctioning of the premises' alarm system. Few of them will ever have encountered expressions such as 'drawings', 'quarterly returns' and 'capital allowances'. The concept of a fee-for-service for clinical procedures may strike them as bizarre, and even unethical. They will almost certainly feel uncomfortable about charging private fees.

The single encounter most likely to precipitate a state of acute culture shock in the new registrar is the receipt of his or her own copy of the Red Book, and the sensitive trainer will wait for an appropriate moment before making the presentation. But, at some stage, the registrar must begin to come to terms with the fact that he or she will soon cease to be an employee and become an employer, a contractor and a negotiator. This transition brings both rights and responsibilities, and entails a number of new roles. This chapter considers these roles in turn.

The GP as organizer of a complex service

The doctor who comes directly from a secondary-care environment is likely to be either disinterested in, or overwhelmed by, the organizational 'nitty-gritty' of providing an efficient and effective primary-care service. However, it is no accident that research undertaken by GPs, and that undertaken by academic departments of primary care, often appears obsessed with 'administrative' issues, such as appointment systems, referral rates, interruptions during consultations and the technicalities of repeat prescribing, rather than with the signs, symptoms and diseases that are, at least in the hospital specialist's eyes, the core material of general practice.

Those who have experience of the undifferentiated and un-filtered nature of primary care know that the art of general practice is crucially concerned with 'managing' the contacts between patients and professionals for episodes of real or perceived illness. Successful primary care is about offering an appropriate, acceptable and affordable package of immediate and ongoing care for all manner of presenting problems, from the acute and trivial to the chronic and incurable. An essential part of that management is manipulating both one's own availability and the patient's access to investigations and specialist care in order to encourage and support self-management, ensure equity of access to expensive resources, and give priority to the sickest, most treatable cases over the vocal and demanding.

Delivering the lesson that good primary care is defined in terms of process as well as content is not easy for the trainer. The new recruit to general practice will have passed a significant mile-stone when he or she has grasped this essential difference between the world of primary care and that of more disease-orientated specialties.

The GP as independent contractor to the health authority

In the run-up to the 1966 Charter, GPs fought successfully to retain the status of independent contractors to, rather than employees of, the health authorities (Eversley, 1997), and have guarded that independent status jealously ever since. The crucial features of this contractual relationship are:

- It is not the remit of health authority staff to tell GPs how to practise (although from April 1999, health authorities are charged with overseeing clinical governance in general practice (Secretary of State for Health, 1997; Scally & Donaldson, 1998)).
- The administrative and financial responsibility of running the practice, including providing premises, staff and equipment, belongs to the GP.
- With few exceptions, GPs are not paid a salary but have a variable income made up from a number of sources (see Table 11.1).

Table 11.1 Examples of fees and allowances that make up the GP's gross NHS income.

Item	Definition	Comment
Basic practice allowance (BPA)	A fixed fee, payable to all GPs with over 400 patients on their list, and rising with broad band of list size up to a maximum payable when list size reaches 1200	In practice, virtually all full-time GPs receive the full basic practice allowance
Capitation fee	A fee per head of registered population, rising with broad band of age such that the over-65s and over-75s attract higher payments	The proportion of intended net remuneration that should be derived from capitation rather than BPA is controversial. Some argue that reducing BPA as a proportion of GMS creates a perverse incentive for excessively high list sizes
Item-of-service fee	A flat fee payable for provision of certain defined services	For example, new registration medicals, minor surgery, out-of-hours visits
Target payments	A lump sum payable on achieving a defined coverage of the eligible practice population	The full 'target fee' is payable on immunization of 90% of infants or undertaking cervical smears on 80% of women with an intact uterus aged 20–64. A smaller sum is payable on achieving lower targets of 70% and 50%, respectively

Trainer's allowance	A stipend for GPs who have completed the required training and currently have an attached registrar
Health-promotion fee	A lump sum for provision of particular health-promotion services, particularly in the field of cardiovascular disease prevention	Often provided on the basis of locally determined contracts negotiated between the practice and the health authority
Disease management fee	A lump sum for provision and/or co-ordination of non-core services for diabetes and asthma	Contracts may be negotiated locally between GPs and health authorities
Fee for non-core services	A fee per registered eligible head of population for provision of non-core GMS services	For example, developmental checks for children under 5, contraceptive services
Postgraduate education allowance (PGEA)	A payment (or part pro rata) in return for evidence that the GP has attended 30 hours of approved educational activity in the previous 12 months	GP principals in the 12 months after completing the registrar year receive the full PGEA

The advantage of independent contractor status, at least in theory, is that it gives GPs more freedom to provide a service that is personal, flexible and responsive to local needs. In addition, it potentially allows the hard-working and well-organized members of the profession to earn considerably more than the average net remuneration. Furthermore, the tax advantages of being 'self-employed' are said to amount to around £800 per full-time partner per year because of the ability to offset expenses against taxable income.

One potential disadvantage of independent contractor status is that the line between legitimate **flexibility** in the organization and delivery of services and unacceptable **variability** in standards of care is not always easy to draw. Having free rein to run one's own show at best fosters innovative and imaginative service developments and appropriate solutions to local problems. However, at worst it fails to constrain poor practice and converts a profession into a commercial enterprise. Financial rewards for particular defined services can create a perverse incentive for GPs to provide unnecessary, inappropriate or duplicated care, as was evidenced by the rise and fall of health-promotion clinics between 1991 and 1994.

In addition, much has been written about the vulnerability of GPs in under-resourced inner-city areas. These practitioners find themselves penalized rather than rewarded for struggling with low list sizes, mobile populations, high levels of morbidity and socioeconomic deprivation, adverse demographic features, such as a high proportion of elderly living alone, poor premises and fear of crime. Attempts to compensate for this multiple jeopardy through differential capitation fees depending on patients' age and a proxy measure of socioeconomic status have partially, but not fully, addressed this problem (Pringle & Morton-Jones, 1994; Lloyd *et al.*, 1995).

Nevertheless, GPs believe that, on balance, both they and their patients benefit from a contractual, rather than an employer–employee, relationship between themselves and the health authority. In 1986, the Conference of Local Medical Committees overwhelmingly rejected the notion of a salaried service with a good practice allowance in favour of retaining independent contractor status.

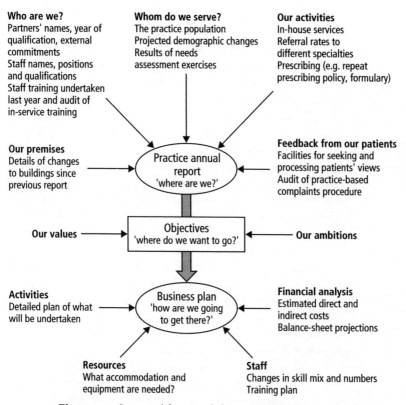

Who are we?
Partners' names, year of qualification, external commitments
Staff names, positions and qualifications
Staff training undertaken last year and audit of in-service training

Whom do we serve?
The practice population
Projected demographic changes
Results of needs assessment exercises

Our activities
In-house services
Referral rates to different specialties
Prescribing (e.g. repeat prescribing policy, formulary)

Our premises
Details of changes to buildings since previous report

Practice annual report
'where are we?'

Feedback from our patients
Facilities for seeking and processing patients' views
Audit of practice-based complaints procedure

Our values

Objectives
'where do we want to go?'

Our ambitions

Activities
Detailed plan of what will be undertaken

Business plan
'how are we going to get there?'

Financial analysis
Estimated direct and indirect costs
Balance-sheet projections

Resources
What accommodation and equipment are needed?

Staff
Changes in skill mix and numbers
Training plan

Figure 11.1 Suggested framework for practice annual report and business plan.

Since 1990, it has been a statutory requirement for GPs to submit an annual report to the health authority, giving details of the practice and the population it serves. A framework for such a report is given in Fig. 11.1.

The GP as director of a small business

Whatever one's higher motives, it is impossible to run any small business without close attention to cash flow. The GP (or, increasingly these days, the executive partner along with the practice manager) must play the role of company bookkeeper and, to this end, must have a clear understanding of both sides of the cash-flow equation, i.e.:

Where does the money come from?

and

What do I have to pay out?

The first of these questions requires an understanding of the broader aspects of NHS finance as well as familiarity with the particular claim forms and quarterly returns of general practice. The second question includes issues of partners' drawings, payments to employed staff, payments involved in running the premises, and tax. While it takes years for the uninitiated to become fully competent in these areas, the aspiring GP should aim to acquire a general understanding of the field by the end of the registrar year. Important areas for discussion are suggested below.

The kitty of money raised by taxation and allocated by the government to spending on health care through the NHS is officially divided into two main categories:

1 Capital money, which is defined as money spent on anything costing over £5000 which has a lifetime of over 1 year, comprises land, buildings and large items of equipment.

2 Revenue money, which is allocated to pay for patient care and is spent largely on wages and consumables, such as drugs, bandages and small items of equipment.

The allocation and expenditure of capital money in the NHS is a fascinating issue. Detailed analysis is outside the scope of this chapter, but the subject is covered in more detail in the references given at the end of this chapter (see in particular Chisolm, 1990; British Medical Association, 1996; Ellis & Chisolm, 1997). From the GP's point of view, capital money becomes available from time to time in the form of invitations to bid for improvement grants to develop practice premises or purchase major pieces of equipment. These funds tend to be administered through the health authority. It should be noted that public funding for capital developments in the NHS have been greatly reduced over the last few years and there is now an increased emphasis on obtaining these resources from the private sector.

Revenue money in the NHS is further divided into:

• Hospital and Community Health Service (HCHS) funds, designated, respectively, for the services provided by hospitals and community trusts.

- Funds administered by health authorities, which comprise General Medical Service (GMS) funds as well as smaller budgets for dental, pharmacy and ophthalmic services in the community.

The entire NHS revenue budget is cash limited (this means that once the allocation has been spent no further resources are available in any one year). The current situation (which many believe is set to change) is that HCHS funds are cash-limited, but GMS funds are non-cash-limited. Thus, for example, drugs supplied to patients in the context of acute hospital care will be paid for only up to a set spending limit, whereas the costs of drugs prescribed on a form FP10 (GP prescription form) will, in theory, be met whatever the cost. Note, however, that the cost of GP prescribing is a subject of major concern both nationally and locally, and a number of pressures and incentives are in place to curtail this potentially limitless use of resources. The 1997 White Paper suggests that the budget for most GP prescribing will become cash-limited from 1999 (Secretary of State for Health, 1997).

As explained above, GPs, as independent contractors, are not paid a salary. The broad limits of their income are set by an independent body appointed by government, who decide annually what the **intended net remuneration** from GMS funds should be per full-time GP partner. This remuneration, multiplied by the number of full-time equivalent GPs, is the amount the government would be required to allocate from GMS funds for this purpose (Ellis & Chisolm, 1997). Using this overall intended net remuneration, and with attention to the 1990 GP Contract, payment levels for fees and allowances are negotiated each year by the General Medical Services Committee (GMSC) of the BMA with the Department of Health. The main fees and allowances are listed in Table 11.1.

From the **gross** income derived from the fees and allowances in Table 11.1, the GP must meet all practice expenses before paying tax on the profits, although the health authority reimburses certain additional costs, including a (negotiable) proportion of staff salaries, computer equipment and certain premises expenditure. The details of such reimbursements are complex and tend to change every year or two. The registrar does not have to commit these details to memory and the details do not feature in the

MRCGP examination—only the general principles need to be understood. However, up-to-date reference texts, such as *Making Sense of the Red Book* (Ellis & Chisolm, 1997) and the GMSC document *Defining Core Services* (General Medical Services Committee, 1997), are essential pieces of surgery equipment.

The proportion of gross income that remains after practice expenses have been paid is the GP's **net** remuneration. The Review body's target for intended average net remuneration in 1997/8 was £47 000.

It should be made clear to the registrar that, whereas the basic practice allowance and capitation fees are **paid automatically** every quarter, claims for the various additional fees and allowances listed in Table 11.1 must be **submitted** to the health authority on a quarterly basis. Every health authority has examples of practices that lose thousands of pounds every year through missed claims as a result of tardiness or administrative inefficiency.

The GP as strategic planner

Textbooks and templates on how to formulate a business plan for general practice are now ubiquitous, but the more fundamental lesson for the GP in training is **why** such a plan is desirable. Winston Churchill said people do not plan to fail, but they do fail to plan. Disputes between partners, disappointments in personal achievements and poor staff communication and commitment may all arise from a lack of a clear, shared set of objectives and priorities and a misunderstanding of everyone's contribution to the team effort.

While business planning will not itself abolish conflict, confusion or underperformance, in practices where the process is taken seriously it is usually perceived as an important contributor to the efficient running of the practice and a vital tool in achieving specific goals set by partners and staff. It should also be noted that, these days, successful applications for development funding rarely occur in the absence of a clearly presented strategy in the shape of a business plan.

As Fig. 11.1 shows, the business plan should stem from a systematic analysis of the practice's current position and activities, and link this reflective process with future goals through a detailed proposal of who needs to do what, when, how and with what resources. For a more detailed perspective on business planning for general practice, see Edwards *et al.* (1994).

The GP as employer

Newcomers to a large practice can find the number and range of staff who work on the premises, and who are apparently part of 'the team', confusing. It might be helpful to provide the new registrar with a framework into which names, faces and roles can be slotted over the year's attachment. Such a framework, looked at from the viewpoint of the GP as employer, might be drawn up as follows:

1 Partners in the practice, who may include:
   • full- and part-time profit-sharing principals
   • salaried GP partners
   • unusually, non-GP partners (for example, practice nurses or managers with a share in the business assets and a profit-sharing agreement).

2 Salaried staff paid by the partnership, who may include:
   • assistants, locums and other doctors who are not part of the partnership
   • practice nurses
   • practice counsellors and psychologists
   • receptionists, managers, secretaries.

3 Attached staff employed by other agencies but working partly or wholly on the practice premises, who may include:
   • district nurses, health visitors, school nurses, physiotherapists, clinical medical officers, midwives, treatment-room nurses and phlebotomists employed by the community trust
   • social workers employed by the local social services department
   • visiting 'outreach' staff, such as hospital consultants, ultrasonographers, etc.

4 Voluntary or private-sector staff, who may include:
   • 'Macmillan' nurses (but note that the organization and funding of community-based terminal care varies with locality)
   • representatives of charities, for example voluntary advocacy services, Jewish Care, National Childbirth Trust, etc.

- private therapists who rent space in the building, for example sports physiotherapists, private-sector GPs.

The employment of staff is governed by common law (i.e. based on legal cases) and statute law (i.e. based on specific Acts of Parliament). Where common law and statute are in conflict, statute prevails.

The duties of an employer under common law are:

1 To provide work. If the failure to provide work leads to a reduction in an employee's actual or potential earnings, the employer will be in breach of the implied term in the contract. Thus, for example, offering sessional work to a counsellor on a fee-per-patient basis and then failing to refer patients would put the partners in breach of the law.

2 To pay wages in return for the employee's work or willingness to be available for work. Thus, if receptionists or secretaries have turned up for work as agreed in a verbal or written contract, and there is insufficient work to occupy them, wages must still be paid.

3 To take reasonable care for the safety of employees. Note that employees must accept some personal responsibility to protect and defend themselves from injury and accidents. As an example, the partners might be reasonably required to provide no-touch phlebotomy systems and adequate 'sharps' boxes, as well as training for staff in the disposal of sharps. However, the partners would not necessarily be found negligent if a properly trained nurse sustained a needlestick injury in the course of his or her work.

4 To indemnify employees for injury sustained while in the employer's service. In practice, this requires the partners to take out comprehensive employer's liability insurance under the advice of a solicitor.

5 To be reasonable in maintaining the employment relationship by treating employees with due consideration and respect. This implied duty has been incorporated into statute law and the regulations on fair and unfair dismissal.

This list of rights and duties is rarely referred to by the naïve employer until problems arise—most commonly in relation to perceived underperformance in an employee. However, it is important to realize that there are numerous reasons for poor performance at work, not all of which relate to individual attitudes

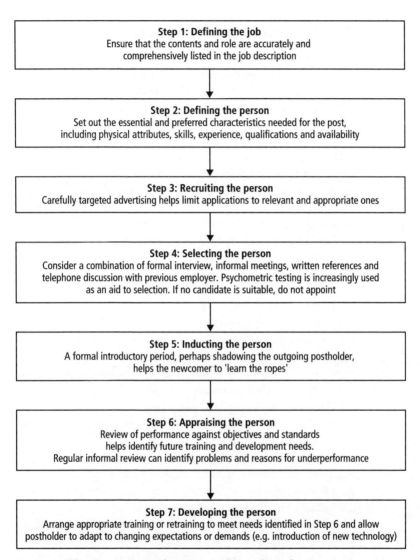

Step 1: Defining the job
Ensure that the contents and role are accurately and
comprehensively listed in the job description

Step 2: Defining the person
Set out the essential and preferred characteristics needed for the post,
including physical attributes, skills, experience, qualifications and availability

Step 3: Recruiting the person
Carefully targeted advertising helps limit applications to relevant and appropriate ones

Step 4: Selecting the person
Consider a combination of formal interview, informal meetings, written references and
telephone discussion with previous employer. Psychometric testing is increasingly used
as an aid to selection. If no candidate is suitable, do not appoint

Step 5: Inducting the person
A formal introductory period, perhaps shadowing the outgoing postholder,
helps the newcomer to 'learn the ropes'

Step 6: Appraising the person
Review of performance against objectives and standards
helps identify future training and development needs.
Regular informal review can identify problems and reasons for underperformance

Step 7: Developing the person
Arrange appropriate training or retraining to meet needs identified in Step 6 and allow
postholder to adapt to changing expectations or demands (e.g. introduction of new technology)

Figure 11.2 Essential steps in avoiding underperformance.

and behaviour. Many arise through lack of attention to detail
in defining the job, in selecting candidates, in giving necessary
appraisal and training and in developing and supporting the person in the work environment (Fig. 11.2).

The GP as a commissioner of services

Prior to the introduction of GP fundholding in 1991, all secondary care was commissioned and paid for through health authorities, and GPs had no direct say in what services were provided. The 1989 White Paper *Working for Patients* (Secretaries of State for Health of Wales, Northern Ireland and Scotland, 1989) heralded the era of the 'primary-care-led NHS'. In the primary-care-led NHS, GPs, as advocates for patients and those most in touch with the needs of local communities, would have an increasing say in what services were provided, as well as in where and how they were provided. The preliminary ideas stated (and implied) in *Working for Patients* were further developed in a number of subsequent Department of Health publications (NHS Executive, 1994; Ministry of Health, 1996; Secretary of State for Health, 1996, 1997).

The principle of GP fundholding was that GP practices would hold a budget to purchase certain services for their patients and negotiate contracts with providers to ensure that these services meet certain specifications. Budgets previously held by the health authority would be devolved to practice level for either:
- Standard fundholding: most hospital procedures (excluding emergencies) and community services.
- Community fundholding: community services (district nurses, health visitors), direct-access physiotherapy and diagnostic tests.
- Total purchasing: all services.

The introduction of fundholding was controversial. Some commentators claimed that fundholding was an effective spur to the improvement of services across the board. However, others claimed that it produced little more than an increase in bureaucracy and a two-tier system of care in which the patients of fundholders are offered more comprehensive, faster or more flexible care than those of non-fundholders. It has also been argued that fundholding budgets, set on the basis of historical spending combined (latterly) with a weighted capitation formula, were overgenerous. A major criticism was that the system was not adequately evaluated before being introduced. For further reading on the fundholding debate, see the publications by the Audit Commission (1996), Glenerster *et al.* (1996) and Singer (1997).

In the 1997 White Paper *The New NHS* (Secretary of State for Health, 1997), the government presented a bold plan for setting up primary-care groups, to be operational from April 1999. It is envisaged that such groups will comprise GP practices and community nurses, and will cover populations of about 100 000. They will replace current forms of commissioning, including GP fundholding. Four possible models are proposed, ranging from a minimum level of involvement to full trust status:

1 Advising health authorities on commissioning.
2 Managing devolved budgets.
3 Independent primary-care trusts responsible for some devolved commissioning.
4 Primary-care trusts responsible for commissioning all primary and secondary care except specialist services.

The New NHS suggests that primary-care groups will move towards a unified budget for commissioning, prescribing and practice administration, with the facility for transferring funds between these different areas of expenditure. There are no plans to unite the purchasing budget with that for GMS services or to remove independent contractor status (Butler & Roland, 1998).

As a preliminary step towards primary-care groups, a number of intermediate models of locality commissioning came into operation in 1998. In some areas, groups of GPs representing 20–40 practices have been allocated a budget to commission all the health care within their locality. These commissioning groups are charged with negotiating 3–5-year service-level agreements (SLAs) with their local providers of services. This process is believed to have fewer transaction costs than GP fundholding while still allowing GPs direct involvement in the commission of services.

At the time of writing, the development of primary-care commissioning groups is still at the pilot stage. However, a number of theoretical options have been given an enthusiastic welcome (see in particular Smith *et al.*, 1996; Singer, 1997), and many GPs are waiting with interest to see if a workable formula can be achieved for their own involvement in commissioning services for patients.

Box 11.1 Example of a letter of complaint

27 Long Lane
Oakwood
Borsetshire

20th July

Dear Dr Goodman

I am writing to complain about the way I was treated by your practice.

Last week my 3-year-old son had a temperature in the night. It was at least 102° and he was screaming with it. I rang the surgery number and got a locum doctor who didn't know us at all, and said just sponge him down, etc. Then in the morning I called the surgery again saying it is **urgent** since his temperature was still up and the lady said well the doctor's very busy and you aren't the only patient on the list you know. She also said it wasn't serious because he didn't have a rash and to shine a light in his eyes which I did.

I was offered an appointment at 11.45 but that would have been another 3 hours so I went to casualty. Then (after **another** long wait) the doctor saw him and did lots of tests and said he was alright.

I am very upset that your receptionist would not let me speak to you and she made me feel totally neurotic, and anyway do they have the training to tell you it isn't serious (e.g. meningitis) when they are really only there to answer the phone.

I hope you will have the time to reply to this letter which could save another child's life.

Yours sincerely

Mrs Tracey Black

Tutorial exercise 1: What issues of practice organization are raised in this letter, and how would you respond to the letter?

Tutorial checklist

By the end of his or her year's attachment, your registrar should be able to address the following tasks (each of which might form the basis for a tutorial and/or assignment):

- Appoint, induct and appraise a new secretary.
- Sort out maternity-leave arrangements for a practice nurse.
- Deal with a complaint about a member of staff who is allegedly rude to patients (see Box 11.1).
- Present 'the books' to the practice accountant.
- Chair a practice meeting.
- Write the practice annual report for the health authority.
- Draft a practice development plan with a view to providing an extended range of services.
- Contribute to a debate among local GP practices about whether to volunteer for a pilot scheme of locality commissioning.

References

Audit Commission (1996) *What the Doctor Ordered: A Study of GP Fundholding in England and Wales*. HMSO, London.

British Medical Association (1996) *Financing the NHS: A Discussion Paper*. BMA, London.

Butler, T. & Roland, M. (1998) How will primary care groups work? *British Medical Journal* **316**, 214–215.

Chisolm, J. (1990) Improving surgery accommodation. In: *Making Sense of the New Contract* (eds N. Ellis & J. Chisolm), pp. 131–146. Radcliffe Medical Press, Oxford.

Edwards, P., Jones, S. & Williams, S. (1994) *Business and Health Planning for General Practice*. Radcliffe Medical Press, Oxford.

Ellis, N. & Chisolm, J. (eds) (1997) *Making Sense of the Red Book*, 3rd edn. Radcliffe Medical Press, Oxford.

Eversley, J. (1997) The 1990 GP contract in context. In: *Making Sense of the Red Book* (eds N. Ellis & J. Chisolm), 3rd edn, pp. 1–14. Radcliffe Medical Press, Oxford.

General Medical Services Committee (1997) *Defining Core Services*. GMSC, London.

Glenerster, H., Cohen, A. & Bovell, V. (1996) *Alternatives to Fundholding*. Discussion paper WSP/123. London School of Economics, London.

Lloyd, D.C., Harris, C.M. & Clucas, D.W. (1995) Low income scheme index: a new deprivation scale based on prescribing in general practice. *British Medical Journal* **310**, 165–169.

Ministry of Health (1996) *Primary Care: The Future. The Listening Process*. Department of Health, London.

NHS Executive (1994) *Developing NHS Purchasing and GP Fundholding. Towards a Primary Care-led NHS*. NHS Executive, Leeds.

Pringle, M. & Morton-Jones, A. (1994) Using unemployment rates to predict prescribing trends in England. *British Journal of General Practice* **44**, 53–56.

Scally, G. & Donaldson, L. (1998) Clinical governance and the drive for quality improvement in the new NHS in England. *British Medical Journal* **317**, 61–65.

Secretaries of State for Health of Wales, Northern Ireland and Scotland (1989) *Working for Patients*. HMSO, London.

Secretary of State for Health (1996) *Primary Care: the Future. Choice and Opportunity*. Department of Health, London.

Secretary of State for Health (1997) *The New NHS: Modern, Dependable*. Department of Health, London.

Singer, R. (ed.) (1997) *GP Commissioning: An Inevitable Evolution*. Radcliffe Medical Press, Oxford.

Smith, R., Butler, F. & Powell, M. (1996) *Total Purchasing: A Model for Locality Commissioning*. Radcliffe Medical Press, Oxford.

12 The trainer

The role of the trainer

What do racehorses, fitness fanatics and delegates on management courses have in common? The answer (too easy perhaps) is, of course, trainers. Trainers can be many things and are, more often than not, several of them at once. Their role varies with time, place, circumstance and whatever their trainee is up to at the time. Trainees in general practice have, since 1995, been officially known as **registrars**, but a more appropriate title has yet to replace the term 'trainer'. We are stuck with the athletic connotations. Training implies some standardized end-product or goal, such as being able to hit a backhand passing shot with top spin or to execute an immaculate pirouette. It can also be defined as a series of exercises or experiences to which a trainee is subjected. Under the general entry 'train', the Collins English Dictionary (1979) also wryly suggests the following definitions: 'to improve or curb by subjecting to discipline, to focus or bring to bear, and a line of gunpowder leading to an explosive charge!' But what exactly is a trainer and what is his or her role? The nub of this chapter—in the context of vocational training—is the theme of this book.

Box 12.1 summarizes the many parts that the trainer is required to play throughout the registrar year and this chapter explores each of them in turn. A brief discussion follows of the place of the trainer in the general-practice educational hierarchy. Then the various ways in which trainers might receive support and the reasons why trainers become trainers in the first place are considered.

Employer

The trainer has the same basic responsibilities to his or her registrar as he or she does to the rest of the employed staff. The details

---

Box 12.1 The roles of the trainer

- Employer
- Supervisor
- Educator
- Assessor
- Role model
- Friend and adviser
- Counsellor
- Advocate
- Referee
- Colleague

Box 12.2 Employment responsibilities of the trainer

- Salary and car allowance to be paid monthly
- Superannuation to be deducted appropriately
- Both parties to be members of a medical defence organization
- Workload imposed not to exceed the average practice workload
- Five weeks' holiday per annum or pro rata
- 30 days of approved study leave
- Full sick pay
- Proper service and educational cover to be arranged when the trainer is on leave
- Trainer to provide the registrar with necessary medical equipment and supplies
- Trainer to be aware of his/her obligations under the vocational training regulations

---

of employment law are concisely summarized elsewhere (Irvine & Haman, 1993), but some of the more important employment issues relating to training are summarized in Box 12.2. The conditions of employment must be set down in a written contract, and an excellent model designed specifically for trainers and their registrars can be obtained through the British Medical Association.

There are other responsibilities too. The trainer is expected to assist the registrar in claiming entitlements laid down in paragraph 38 of the Statement of Fees and Allowances (the 'Red Book'). These may include:

- House-removal expenses.
- Installation of a telephone extension.
- Losses incurred as a consequence of moving to take up a registrar position.
- Miscellaneous expenses, ranging from redirection of mail to alteration of curtain pelmets!

The trainer must also ensure that the registrar is paid appropriately. The salary is calculated on a sliding scale depending on past experience. A car allowance should also be claimed on the registrar's behalf.

Supervisor

Supervision encompasses a range of activities, from policing prescriptions to discussing problems brought to tutorials. Although an independent practitioner, the registrar enters an agreement with the trainer that implies a degree of shared responsibility. It is one of the trainer's hardest tasks. At what point in the year should the registrar be given free rein? Controlled separation and the development of a sense of self-reliance are vitally important in the completion of a successful registrarship, but when the situation is misjudged trainers may be viewed as being mollycoddling or unsupportive. Successful supervision requires ready availability and a keen and watchful eye. The trainer should ensure that well-intentioned actions bring about no harm and that serious mistakes are not made in the first place.

The responsibility of the trainer does not extend to medical negligence and the registrar must be separately insured. Complaints against the registrar which reach the level of the health authority **will** involve the trainer, who can be found in breach of his or her terms of service if the level of supervision provided is deemed inadequate.

Educator

A pedantic term perhaps, but others, 'teacher' and 'tutor' for instance, both have implications that undermine the adult nature of the registrar's learning experience. A tutor is someone in charge of another person's education. As an adult learner the

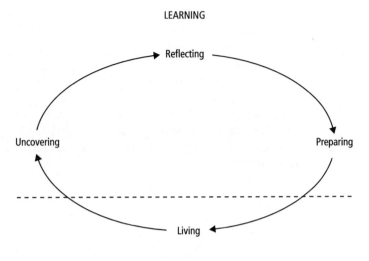

Figure 12.1 The experiential learning cycle.

registrar is very much in charge of his or her own. Teaching can be defined as 'the giving of instruction and the passive receipt of that instruction by the listener'. But adults learn best when there is an intrinsic motivation to learn; when there is a need to connect information already stored. Adult learning tends to be problem centred, arising directly out of experience, and the skill of the trainer in how that experience is meted out, reflected on and interpreted.

The process of experiential learning has been teased apart by many authors including Heron (1976). The learning cycle shown in Fig. 12.1 is typical. The cycle is, of course, in reality a spiral and the whole process of discovery and questioning is a repetitive one, poignantly summarized by the poet T.S. Eliot:

> We shall not cease from exploration
> And the end of all our exploring
> Will be to arrive where we started
> And know the place for the first time.

There are four classical teaching styles that a trainer may adopt in order to facilitate the learning cycle and each impinges on a different zone of the process. A skilled trainer will choose the right moment for each type of intervention, providing information 'in the right way at the right time'. These teaching styles are summarized below:

- Didactic: 'I'll tell you what I know.'

  Essentially a pedagogical style, which has its uses from time to time, usually at the outset of training—'closed certificates can only be written for up to a fortnight'—or in moments of extreme crisis—'1 ml of adrenaline subcutaneously and call an ambulance!'.

- Socratic: 'Tell me what you know.'

  An interrogative style, otherwise known as guided problem solving. Helpful in uncovering deficiencies in knowledge, this rather surgical approach can leave its victim stranded and helpless. Lifelines should be thrown at frequent intervals.

- Heuristic: 'Go and find out and come back and tell me.'

  The learner is trained to discover things for himself. Evidence-based medicine in its purest form, as propounded by Sackett *et al.* (1996), is a good example.

- Counselling: 'How do you feel about it?'

  A facilitative intervention which enables the learner to explore the problem and hopefully arrive at a solution.

  Teaching styles and methods are discussed in more detail in Chapters 3 and 4.

The educational contract

These educational methods will be alien to a newly arrived registrar, perhaps more used to picking up didactic scraps thrown to the floor during consultant ward rounds. Adult learning requires a commitment from the individual and, in order to set things off on the right track, many trainers use an educational contract. This agreement, ideally negotiated at the outset of training, is intended to make clear the aims and objectives of the attachment. It should also outline the induction arrangements and discuss the learning, teaching and assessment methods that are to be used. Foreman (1997) provides a comprehensive list of possible contents and suggests some structures for such a contract. The document is of even more value if the trainer and registrar collaborate in its construction.

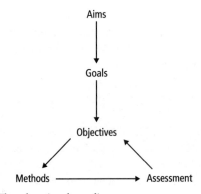

Figure 12.2 The educational paradigm.

Assessor

The traditional educational paradigm (see Fig. 12.2) will be familiar to all teachers and trainers and assessment forms a crucial part of it. Summative assessment has been covered elsewhere in this book (see Chapters 7 and 10) and has, over recent years, taken the focus away from day-to-day assessment methods. These **formative assessment** tools (see Box 12.3) help registrars plan what they need to learn next and give both parties in the educational dyad an idea about their overall progress through the general practice curriculum.

Role model

Some may feel uncomfortable with this role, but like it or not, trainers have a profound influence on registrars just by being who they are and doing things in the way in which they do them. The experience can work either way around, and negative modelling can also occur, when the registrar takes active steps to avoid behaviours exhibited by his or her trainer. Unfortunately, role modelling is a two-edged sword and bad habits are as readily picked up as good. Trainers must be careful about the way they perform when giving demonstrations or when registrars are sitting in. 'Do as I say, not as I do' was never a very effective educational maxim.

Box 12.3 Formative assessment tools

- MCQs
- Modified essay questions
- Project
- Audit
- Personality profiles
- Consultation observation, e.g. video taping, joint surgeries
- 'Hot' topics
- Prescription analysis
- Confidence rating scales
- Follow-up slip system
- Phased evaluation programmes
- Logbook
- Registrar's rolling assessment diary
- Simulated surgeries
- Attitude questionnaires
- Random- and problem-case analysis

A detailed description of these tools and methods (Rhodes, 1994) is available from the Department of Postgraduate General Practice, North Thames (West)

Friend and adviser

This is an extremely important role, which can involve anything from recharging car batteries to making a video film at weddings and advising on cot mattresses. Trainers and registrars often remain firm and lasting friends. However, the relationship sometimes does not click and, while this does not necessarily mean that the training period will be dysfunctional, it doesn't help. Conversely, the danger of an overfriendly relationship is the emergence of collusion, the avoidance of confrontation and the consequent missing out on educational opportunities.

Counsellor

The training year is a turbulent one. It is commonly a time for moving house, putting down roots and making important decisions about careers, marriages and births. It is also the first chance that the registrar, processed through the academic mill of 'A' levels, medical school, house-officer posts and the vocational training scheme, has had to take stock. Indeed, many registrars having arrived at this stage feel they need longer to think over their future. This is often a time when a career break is taken, perhaps involving working abroad or starting a family. A partnership position is potentially a job for life—a daunting prospect when your former time unit of permanence has been 6 months. Such a change may cause a considerable amount of stress, anxiety and even depression, and many trainers find themselves having to cope with a distracted registrar in emotional turmoil. Maintaining an academic impetus through this obstacle course of life events can be near impossible, and sometimes it is simply better to give up, support the registrar through the immediate crisis and await the next opportunity to re-engage. Counselling, whether advisory, supportive or catalytic, can be a real help to registrars at this time but occasionally severe stress can give rise to serious mental health problems. In this instance, the trainer is advised not to add physician or indeed psychotherapist to his or her already confused list of roles. No one benefits from this degree of enmeshment and the impartial help of a colleague should be sought.

Advocate

The early days can be daunting for the newly arrived registrar, who is attempting to make an impression on a bunch of seasoned receptionists, a busy partnership and distant hospital consultants, not to mention the blue blur of frenetic district nurses. A good trainer will soon connect up his or her registrar with the practice, the hospital and the primary-care team, but the trainer also has a role in the maintenance of these connections. General practice is about long-term relationships and registrars in their first few months, some throughout their training, can appear gauche, shy, uncommunicative, overconfident or just downright rude. Often these teething problems arise from the misjudgement of people and situations or may simply indicate a lack of awareness of local history and associated psychodynamics. The trainer's job in the role as advocate is to pour oil on troubled waters, to extol the virtues of his or her apprentice and to kindle relationships which will help the registrar grow throughout his or her time in the practice.

Advocacy sometimes also extends to more gruelling tasks, such as attending service hearings, appealing against summative assessment decisions, arranging periods of further training and, more positively, finding the registrar a partnership...

Referee

... the first stage of which is **the reference**. Often a pleasure, occasionally a source of dread, one's name on the bottom of the registrar's CV is one of the final responsibilities of the trainer. How easy it is to write a good reference and how difficult to write a bad one. Candid objectivity is hard to find when you have nurtured your young colleagues, taught them everything that you know (and hopefully more!), counselled them through various family crises and become their friend. Any sensible future employer would not ask a trainer for a reference in the first place!

Colleague

The transition from pupil to colleague is gradual and proceeds slowly throughout the training year. The relationship builds on mutual respect and focuses around the adoption of a set of professional values that distinguish the 9-to-5 jobbing doctor from the vocational physician. Many registrars remain as partners in the practice in which they trained and most stay within the area, becoming colleagues in neighbouring practices. The critical time for this transition occurs towards the end of the training year and will be greatly facilitated if an 18-month training period becomes standard. One proposal for the structuring of this additional time refers to 'senior registrars', who will have survived the ordeal of summative assessment and sat the membership examination of the Royal College of General Practitioners (MRCGP). They can then prepare themselves for the increased workload and different ways of working that distinguish the experience of the registrar in his or her final months from that of the newly appointed partner.

The special relationship that exists between trainer and registrar continues long after training has been completed, and many apprentices still turn to their 'sorcerers' for help and advice throughout their career.

Part-time training

Many trainers have to fulfil other roles outside the practice (such as parent for instance) which only permit them to train on a part-time basis. A recent European Union directive (93/16/EEC) has stipulated that a part-time registrar should have a weekly training commitment of at least 60% of that of a full-time colleague. This poses a problem for any trainer intending to work half-time. Training is considered complete after 20 months, provided that it has included some experience (duration unspecified) of full-time work.

The hierarchy of educational responsibility

The organization of postgraduate medical education has undergone considerable change in the last few years and remains in a state of flux. There is considerable variation around the country and the best one can do at the present time is to paint a generalized picture of who a trainer might relate to in an idealized region. A hierarchical tree is shown in Fig. 12.3. Recommendations on general-practice training are currently made to regions by the Joint Committee on Postgraduate Training for General Practice (JCPTGP), who are also the watchdog organization inspecting regions for the quality of their training arrangements. The JCPTGP is, in addition, the body responsible for issuing **certificates of satisfactory completion**.

One of the more recent innovations in medical educational politics is the setting up of local educational boards. On these sit representatives of all stakeholders in postgraduate general-practice education, including not only trainers, course organizers and general-practice tutors but also members of the health authority, the medical audit advisory group, the local RCGP faculty and the local medical committee. Co-ordination of postgraduate general-practice medical education may yet be achieved!

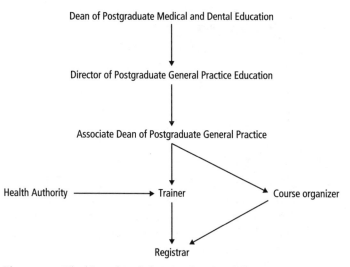

Figure 12.3 The hierarchy of educational responsibility.

Support is available for a trainer from a variety of sources, but his or her immediate line manager is the associate dean for the area, although in some smaller regions he or she will report directly to the Director of Postgraduate General Practice Education. Other sources of support include the local trainers' workshop, course organizers, fellow trainers and the education division of the RCGP. Publications such as *Education for General Practice* and the *British Journal of General Practice* may provide a sounding-board and events such as trainers' conferences and regional trainers' days allow networking and the exchange of problems and ideas.

The trainers' workshop

Attendance at a trainers' workshop is a mandatory requirement for trainer reapproval. Stipulations vary from region to region but typically trainers are required to attend two-thirds of the sessions of a workshop, which in turn is expected to meet for 2 hours each month. This is quite a commitment. Workshops are also considered by the JCPTGP to be part of the remunerated work of the trainer and therefore not eligible for the Postgraduate Education Allowance.

Box 12.4 Functions of a trainers' workshop

- News and information
- Trainer support network
- Teaching exchange
- Problem sharing
- Link with vocational training scheme
- Continuing trainer education

Trainers' workshops fulfil many functions (see Box 12.4) and are attended with varying degrees of enthusiasm. In common with any group, a cycle of formation, growth and senescence dictates the vibrancy and cohesiveness of the group at any one time. The workshop is a forum for the airing of problems, concerns and practical difficulties, as well as providing an opportunity for trainers to learn together and develop their educational knowledge and skills. The workshop also provides a vital link with the local course organizers and facilitates the distribution of registrars among the participating trainers.

Innovative trainers' workshops are in existence up and down the country. Some have focused their efforts on producing research papers, others have become involved in mentoring and portfolio learning schemes. Trainers, by and large, are an untapped pool of educational expertise and it may well be that their involvement in undergraduate teaching will increase over the next few years, as university medical schools attempt to increase the proportion of community-based teaching on offer. Trainers may also soon find themselves involved in the reaccreditation process, as either assessors, mentors or teachers.

The trainer and the vocational training scheme

The strength of links between trainers and vocational training schemes (VTSs) varies throughout the country. Course organizers are usually ex-trainers and many continue to train while they hold the post. It is customary for them to attend the trainers' workshop and they are responsible for the allocation of registrars to particular trainers. In most regions an agreement is made with registrars that a training placement will be made available to them.

Contracts are drawn up independently between trainers and registrars, and registrars and the VTS.

VTSs can become isolated from the day-to-day business of training and it is important that trainers are kept involved. This can be achieved by inviting trainers to teach on the half-day-release sessions, to joint workshop meetings and to regular social events. A course organizers' slot in the monthly workshop is also useful.

Half-day-release sessions are becoming more educationally accountable. Attendance is a contractual obligation of the registrar. Trainers can encourage the valuing of this important fixture in the weekly schedule by ensuring registrars attend the session on time, covering the registrar's on-call commitments and expressing an interest in what has gone on at the session.

Training problems

Every registrar brings to the trainer a new set of problems. It goes, as they say, with the territory. Many of the difficulties that arise stem directly from the complexity of that relationship and the multifarious and often conflicting roles that the trainer has to play. Help and support are available from a variety of sources. These are illustrated in the following examples, each accompanied by a discussion.

Example 1
In his introductory 3 months in general practice Eric repeatedly demonstrated his incompetence and inability to assimilate new information. His trainer's view was that he should never become a GP and would struggle to pass summative assessment. The hospital consultants had serious concerns too but, not wanting to enter into any confrontation, signed him up, relieved to see him go. As a pre-emptive measure, his prospective trainer decided to bring up the subject of Eric at a trainers' workshop.

Discussion. Not surprisingly, the trainer wants to protect his or her partners, the patients of the practice and him- or herself from substandard and potentially dangerous clinical practice. The trainer does not, of course, have to take Eric on, as a contract will not yet have been signed. Most VTSs are not contractually obliged to place final-year registrars, although there is an implicit agreement that this will take place. If none of the trainers on the scheme will take Eric, then he will have to look elsewhere to complete his training. This effectively plants the problem on someone else's doorstep and Eric's need for high-quality training is arguably greater than most. Summative assessment may eventually prevent his entry into the profession but this sort of problem is best dealt with at an early stage.

In Eric's first 3 months of training, a discussion with the course organizers would have been very useful. The views of the hospital consultants could then have been actively sought and hopefully reflected in more accurate assessments. Eric might then have been offered counselling about possible alternative career paths. This remains the advisable course of action. If he persists with his training, then the workshop needs to discuss who would be best placed to take him, perhaps a trainer in a practice with a lighter workload or someone with special expertise or experience.

Additional training may be helpful and there is provision for health authorities to fund an additional training period of 6 months should an application to the dean of postgraduate general practice meet with approval. Casualties of summative assessment might also avail themselves of this, and in some regions remedial training practices have been proposed. At the time of writing, a target of 18 months' training in general practice for all registrars is being worked towards, but precisely how such a scheme will work, be implemented and be funded is currently the source of much debate.

Example 2

Peter repeatedly phoned in sick, complaining of migraines. He would be off for several days at a time and his surgeries would frequently have to be cancelled at short notice. After 9 months of disruption, partners were furious, patients were frustrated and Peter had lost 6 weeks of his registrar year to date through illness.

Discussion. This is another of those situations that positions the trainer uncomfortably between his or her charge and the partners. However, the partnership may be a useful ally in confronting Peter over his sickness record. The partnership can also insist on such protective measures as only booking Peter's appointments on the day or leaving another partners's surgery half-booked until he has arrived.

As far as sick leave and its impact on training is concerned, periods of up to 2 weeks are generally ignored. Beyond that regions vary in their approach, but most require discussion with the associate dean for the area. Most associate deans will tolerate between 2 and 4 weeks' sick leave, depending on the educational needs and circumstances of the registrar, but this would normally be discussed with the registrar concerned and his or her trainer. Beyond that time, an extension to the training period will be necessary.

Example 3
The receptionists considered Rachael bolshie and uncooperative. Unfortunately, so did the patients and on more than one occasion a complaint had been made to the practice about her. Late in her training year, a particular out-of-hours call had gone unusually badly. Unfortunately, the flu diagnosed by Rachael over the telephone was more accurately identified by the coroner 10 days later as a myocardial infarction. The patient had subsequently died of a presumed ventricular dysrhythmia. The family, angered by the misdiagnosis together with the registrar's attitude, insisted on taking the complaint further.

Discussion. Prevention is better than cure and this is an example where early consultation with the course organizers would have been of value. A joint meeting with Rachael might have addressed some of the attitudinal issues before this crisis point had been reached. Most complaints are made about doctors not well known to individual patients and many of these involve some element of communication breakdown. Confrontational registrars may therefore be particularly vulnerable to complaints.

A complaint made to the practice first passes through 'in-house' procedures. Although the trainer is bound to be consulted early on in proceedings, it is probably more appropriate that the investigating partner is one of his or her colleagues. The complaint can then be discussed more dispassionately and the trainer's role becomes easier, concentrating on support and the educational issues rather than having to stand in judgement at the same time. Should the complaint escalate up to the health authority, trainer and registrar are both very much involved. Issues of adequacy of supervision and availability may be raised and both parties are likely to need support through what can be a harrowing and deeply unsettling experience.

Should the family decide to take legal action, the trainer has no liability. Each doctor is insured against his or her own negligence and every registrar should be a member of a recognized medical defence organization.

Why do trainers train?

This is a simple question to which there is no simple answer. Some small-scale attempts have been made to explore this complex issue. In a recent qualitative study (Spencer Jones, 1997), three broad classes of responses from trainers were identified: trainer-centred, practice-centred and registrar-centred (see Box 12.5). To these I would cynically add *remuneration* and *an extra pair of hands*, although no trainer would dare admit it in public! More altruistically, and perhaps nearer the psychological hub of the

---

Box 12.5 Why do trainers train?

Trainer-centred reasons:
• Intellectually stimulating
• A challenge
• A boost to self-esteem
• Motivated by their own training experience, either positive or negative

Registrar-centred reasons:
• Satisfaction in seeing young doctors develop and grow

Practice-centred reasons:
• Increased self-esteem
• Increased practice esteem
• Practice better organized and more focused
• Increased standing of trainer and practice within the professional community

matter, Zen influenced Neighbour in his book the *Inner Apprentice* (Neighbour, 1992). Neighbour writes of a 'dynastic impulse to show', a need to pass on knowledge, values and our thought processes to the next generation. A concept with which I am sure every parent, and I suspect most trainers, will resonate.

To 'arrive where we started'—what is a trainer? Adult education has been described as a 'transformational journey' (Daloz, 1986), in which master teachers or **mentors** are our guides. Tales of such journeys and their associated mentors permeate our culture from Greek mythology to contemporary children's fiction and these stories help us to understand the accession of knowledge and wisdom. Furthermore, the mentor has been identified as a psychological archetype by the psychoanalyst Carl Jung (Jung, 1958), as a figure representing 'knowledge, reflection, insight, wisdom, cleverness and intuition' appearing where 'insight, understanding, good advice, determination, planning, etc. are needed but cannot be mustered on one's own'.

If the term trainer is ever to be replaced, perhaps the word mentor should be chosen. We all, it seems, need mentors and some, it would appear, have an overwhelming need to become mentors themselves.

References

Daloz, L.A. (1986) *Effective Teaching and Mentoring.* Jossey-Bass, San Francisco.

Foreman, N. (1997) The educational contract kit. *Education for General Practice* **8**, 360–363.

Heron, J. (1976) *Six Category Intervention Analysis.* Human Potential Resource Group, University of Surrey, Guildford.

Irvine, S. & Haman, H. (1993) *Making Sense of Personnel Management.* Radcliffe Medical Press, Oxford.

Jung, C.J. (1958) *Psyche and Symbol.* Doubleday, New York.

Neighbour, R. (1992) *The Inner Apprentice.* Kluwer Academic, London.

Rhodes, M. (ed.) (1994) *Formative Assessment Workbook,* 2nd edn. Department of Postgraduate General Practice, North Thames (West).

Sackett, D.L., Richardson, W.S., Rosenberg, W. & Haynes, R.B. (1996) *Evidence Based Medicine—How to Practice and Teach EBM.* Churchill Livingstone, Edinburgh.

Spencer Jones, R. (1997) Why do trainers train? *Education for General Practice* **8**(1), 31–39.

Further reading

Joint Committee on Postgraduate Training for General Practice (1992) *Recommendations to Regions for the Establishment of Criteria for the Approval and Reapproval of Trainers in General Practice.* JCPTGP, London.

Rosenthal, J., Naish, J. & Lloyd, M. (1994) *The Trainee's Companion to General Practice.* Churchill Livingstone, London.

Royal College of General Practitioners (1994) *Education and Training for General Practice.* RCGP, London.

13   Becoming a trainer

Standards in vocational training

The job of teaching the next generation of doctors is important and privileged. Trainers in general practice are especially fortunate, as teaching is something they can choose to do and for which they are paid specifically. This gives them an advantage over their consultant and academic colleagues, for whom, like it or not, teaching is part of their job and attracts no extra pay. GP trainers are paid a 'training grant', which, in 1998, was £5220 per annum, and GP registrars' salaries are reimbursed in full.

However, this fortunate position has its responsibilities. GP registrars have a right to expect high standards of teaching, clinical medicine and practice organization from their training practices. The following bodies ensure that trainers achieve and maintain these standards:

- The Joint Committee on Postgraduate Training for General Practice (JCPTGP).
- The regional general practice education sub-committees.

The JCPTGP has a statutory duty to monitor vocational training and sends representatives to each deanery every 3 years to ensure that quality in vocational training schemes (VTSs) is being maintained. It publishes a booklet (Joint Committee on Postgraduate Training for General Practice, 1998) setting out its policy on trainer selection and stipulating a number of minimum standards for training practices.

The regional sub-committees have a statutory responsibility for appointing trainers (Department of Health, 1996) and most of them add criteria to reflect local priorities and interests. Additionally, they may stipulate that training practices provide items that are important for training purposes, such as video equipment, disease registers and libraries.

There are three reasons for insisting on high standards in training practices:
- To ensure that registrars receive a professional education programme.
- To ensure that registrars experience a good role model of general practice.
- To prevent exploitation.

These have been described as the 'Three Es'—Education, Example and prevention of Exploitation (A.P. Lewis, personal communication, 1997).

Preparing to become a trainer

GPs who wish to become trainers need to prepare themselves and their practices to meet the high standards necessary. The JCPTGP's booklet is useful reading, but prospective trainers must establish at an early stage the precise criteria they will have to meet. They should obtain a copy of their region's own criteria from the regional adviser's office, as they will be assessed against these criteria.

The JCPTGP booklet sets out the criteria under three headings, and many regions follow a similar format, as it provides a useful framework with which to examine the attributes expected of a trainer. They are:
- The trainer as a clinician.
- The trainer as a teacher.
- The training practice.

The trainer as a clinician

Trainers should have a reasonable amount of experience in general practice. Three years is usually considered the minimum. It would be unwise for doctors to be responsible for teaching others before they feel comfortable with their own skills.

Measuring clinical skill is notoriously difficult, and regions vary in the evidence they require in support of this area of competence. Most now expect new trainers to hold the MRCGP, and some call for video tapes of consultations. Prospective trainers should also be eligible for the postgraduate education allowance (PGEA) and show that they have a thoughtful approach to their own continuing education.

Since 1996 the production of an audit project has been a component of summative assessment and the JCPTGP requires trainers to demonstrate clinical audit to registrars. Trainers might also use audits of clinical work and methodical recording of important clinical and preventive information, such as smoking habits, immunization uptake and blood-pressure reading, as evidence of high clinical standards.

The trainer as a teacher

The ability to teach is the one attribute that separates trainers from their non-training colleagues, irrespective of their other skills. It is likely, therefore, that prospective trainers will need to invest much of their preparation time in this area.

They will need to complete a course for new trainers. Traditionally these have been 5-day residential events, which attempt to cover as much of the material as possible in the time allowed.

This approach has its limitations. Five days away from the home and practice is not always possible, especially for female doctors. (The number of female trainers has not kept pace with the increasing number of women in general practice.) An intensive course also provides little time for reflection, reading and teaching practice. It is also specific to general practice, and trainers may not be able to transfer the skills they learn to any other field of activity, such as adult education or industry.

For these reasons, some regions are looking at alternative formats. The Oxford Region provides a distance learning package, spread over a period of several months, and the South West region offers a certificate of training practice granted by the Institute of Personnel and Development. Perhaps the main outcome of these developments will be that GP trainers become even more professional than they are at present, and that their skills become sought after in areas other than vocational training.

Most VTSs have trainer workshops, where established trainers meet to discuss problems and work on developments in medical education. Potential trainers are usually welcome to join on an informal basis and thereby gain useful insight into the work of a GP trainer.

Potential trainers are expected to be familiar with educational theory, including formative and summative assessment, curriculum planning and teaching methods. They need to show how they will record registrars' progress, problems and achievements. Documentation is especially important, as trainers are increasingly being asked to justify their decisions about their registrars' abilities to practise.

Demonstrating these qualities is difficult for potential trainers, but they should be ready to discuss educational theory and demonstrate that they have available tools, such as assessment packages, logbooks and curriculum plans. Doctors in practices with an established trainer are in a strong position. The practice should already meet the structural requirements, and the current trainer will be able to offer advice on how to meet the other criteria. If there is a registrar in post, they can practise teaching and make a contribution to the training process before being officially approved.

Established trainers can submit documentation relevant to previous registrars. In the South and West established trainers are expected to provide a video of a teaching session as part of their reassessment and this option is also open to new trainers.

The training practice

Future GPs usually obtain their first real experience of general practice in their training practices. These will therefore have a profound influence on their attitude to the discipline and they must offer a first-class role model, with good organization, communications and teamwork, as well as sound clinical medicine.

For these reasons, the quality of the practice features highly in trainer selection. Most training practices have excellent premises with an adequate complement of well-trained staff. Appointment systems should provide reasonable access to doctors and nurses, and be flexible enough to cater for urgent problems and emergencies.

The JCPTGP has always emphasized the importance of good medical records. This includes well-structured record envelopes, with letters and cards tagged together in date order. The clinical history must be summarized and current and past medication clearly identifiable. These are often partly or wholly computerized, and some regions expect registrars to have experience of using computers during consultations.

Registrars must have ready access to current information. Traditionally, trainers have relied on the practice library to provide a selection of books and journals relevant to general practice. However, increasing numbers of training practices have access to MEDLINE and the Internet. This is becoming more important with the growing interest in evidence-based medicine and the emphasis placed on familiarity with current literature in the MRCGP examination.

It is important that the trainer and registrar do not become isolated. The best training practices act as **training units**, with everyone, including all the partners, nurses and managers, involved in providing a stimulating learning environment.

The selection procedure

Each regional sub-committee has its own arrangements for appointing trainers. Whatever the precise form of the procedure, the purpose is threefold:
- To ensure that trainers meet with national and regional criteria.
- To identify areas where improvement is desirable, even when the minimum standard is in place.
- To encourage excellence and innovation.

Selection begins with the potential trainer completing an application form, and is normally followed by a visit to the practice and an interview.

The application form provides an opportunity for potential trainers to demonstrate that they meet the relevant criteria. It would be almost impossible to check every aspect of a practice at one visit, and the initial paperwork allows many of the routine matters to be dealt with beforehand. For example, the form might ask for information about employed staff, the practice library and the organization of the clinical records. Trainers might also be asked to enclose examples of audits, formative assessments and curriculum plans. The onus is on potential trainers to prove that they meet the criteria by providing the necessary evidence.

The purpose of the visit is to examine those aspects of practices that cannot easily be assessed in any other way and to confirm samples of evidence previously submitted. Where practices have registrars in post, they are important witnesses as to the quality of the training. They might draw attention to shortcomings in training, but equally they might identify areas of excellence.

Visiting teams represent the regional advisory committee for general practice education, and their composition depends on regional policy. The JCPTGP recommends that teams should have a broad base and include representatives from course organizers, experienced trainers, clinical tutors, university departments and local medical committees. Normally the teams have three members, led by the regional adviser or his or her representative. There is scope for widening the composition still further; the Oxford Region has included practice managers in its teams and there is a good case for including practice nurses, especially those involved in nurse training.

Trainers naturally find the assessment visit daunting. All assessment is threatening, however much we try to make it part of everyday work and education. Nevertheless, visiting teams are not trying to find fault with the minutiae of practice education or trick trainers into uttering educational heresies. Their aim is to ensure that basic minimum standards are met and, equally important, to encourage excellence. The key to a trouble-free assessment visit is careful preparation.

Approval

Trainers initially receive a maximum of 2 years' approval, and established trainers up to 5 years of reapproval. Most trainers perform extremely well, but those who fail to meet important criteria might have their approval withheld or withdrawn. This is unusual, but, where there is scope or need for improvement, they may receive a reduced period of approval. The figures relating to this in Devon and Cornwall between 1992 and 1997 were:

- Not approved or approval withdrawn—6%.
- Approved but with a reduced period—8%.

The position of GP trainer is important and privileged. Becoming a trainer needs careful preparation in both developing the skills needed to teach and ensuring that the practice meets the requirements. However, the rewards, both financial and in personal satisfaction, are well worth the effort for anyone who wishes to help to maintain the quality of doctors entering general practice.

References

Department of Health (1996) *Statement of Fees and Allowances for General Medical Practitioners in England and Wales*. HMSO, London.

Joint Committee on Postgraduate Training for General Practice (1998) *Recommendations to Deaneries on the Selection and Re-Selection of General Practice Trainers*. JCPTGP, London.

14 Reading and writing

Introduction

Reading and writing research papers are simply two sides of the same skill. When writing, we build a manuscript using a number of key components. When reading, we dissect a paper to expose all these components and assess their quality. These twin skills of reading and writing are becoming increasingly important with the evolution of general practice as an academic discipline. Research is now an established component of general practice, with the recent expansion in the number of academic departments, and research general practices funded outside the university system. Thus, the ability to write a research paper is a key skill, a skill that applies equally to submitting an abstract, an academic presentation or a grant application. Likewise, there is increasing emphasis on the ability to read critically as a fundamental part of practising evidence-based medicine. In this chapter, reading and writing skills will be explored together, and in discussing how to appraise a research paper the basics of writing a paper will be addressed. Critical reading has expanded greatly, so that it covers not just original research but also assessing review articles, economic analyses and qualitative research. This chapter focuses particularly on the original research paper.

Maintaining knowledge

Knowledge drives the decision-making process, but one's knowledge is determined by many factors, including the commitment to continuing medical education, individual strategies for keeping up to date and the availability of information. With the current emphasis on evidence-based practice, there is considerable interest in how doctors seek information, how they evaluate this information and how they apply it in practice.

GPs obtain their information from a variety of sources. Basic medical knowledge comes from undergraduate teaching, but this information is constantly supplemented and updated throughout a medical career. It is unrealistic to expect that the knowledge gained in 3 years of clinical teaching could be adequate to sustain quality medical practice for 40 years—of course it is not.

Knowledge is constantly revised and re-evaluated, but the quality of the revision depends on the quality of the information and the methods used to sort it. New information comes from many sources. Doctors may learn from their experience, but experience is not always a good teacher and may simply reinforce inappropriate behaviour, so that the same mistakes continue to be made with increasing confidence and conviction. Doctors also learn, as do patients, from friends, colleagues and the media. We are not immune to those same factors that influence our patients and we are acutely aware, in our everyday work, of how such messages may be misinterpreted or manipulated. We also learn from drug companies, who inform doctors, through advertising and by visiting representatives, but it must not be forgotten that these companies survive only because their products sell and they invest in advertising and employ representatives because marketing works. These factors all influence our thinking and, while they may be unreliable, we cannot cocoon ourselves and ignore their effect.

We learn from other informal sources too: the hospital letters of referred patients, lectures, discussing case-studies, educational tapes and videos. Further information is available on the Internet and from interactive computer disks. Formal consensus statements, guidelines and protocols, which may appear to have a more scientific basis, are issued by patients' groups, specialist medical organizations and voluntary and statutory bodies. In addition, GPs' postboxes are flooded with a variety of newsletters, magazines and journals. Not only is it impossible to read and digest all of this material, but it is equally difficult to grade the scientific validity of all this information. Listing all these possible sources of information highlights the difficulties involved in keeping up to date. Clearly an information strategy is needed.

Evidence-based medicine

The need to keep up to date and use informed decision making is linked closely with the concept of 'evidence-based medicine', which is discussed fully in Chapter 9.

Reading a research paper demands knowledge of how to search out and evaluate the evidence. We read because we want to keep up to date with the best current treatments and manage our patients most effectively. Decisions to introduce new findings into clinical practice should be determined by the quality of the evidence, but this quality can only be judged if we know how to read, and read effectively. In writing a paper, we build from the introduction and background, move on to address important features of the methodology which determine the quality of the article, and draw together the results and conclusions in a coherent and meaningful way. We write because we have a message, a conclusion or an important new finding that we wish to publish, but the strength of the message is determined by the quality of both the research and the writing.

Learning from reading

When doctors are asked how they keep up to date, they usually say through reading (Smith, 1996). However, what people say they do and what they actually do are not always the same (Covell *et al.*, 1985). Although doctors in the USA (Stinson & Mueller, 1980) and Canada (Curry & Putnam, 1981) claim to read journals for 3 hours per week, it would be difficult for doctors in the UK to do so. It is clearly impossible to digest all the educational material available and it must be approached in some systematic manner. Time is short and we cannot read everything, so we must ruthlessly focus our reading. It is this structured selection, appraisal and digestion of the literature that is critical reading (Jones, 1991). This process has two major components, what and how—what articles to read (and the criteria used in this selection) and how to read articles effectively (and guidelines for assessing their quality).

What to read

It would be impossible to read all the material that is available and, furthermore, not all is of high quality. Some ground rules are needed to direct us to the most appropriate material and to help us select for quality. The volume of literature is overwhelming, and the material worth reading should be sorted from that to be discarded. This may not be easy, and many doctors find themselves frustrated as they try to read everything. Others never start! Before examining methods of reading in detail, it is an idea to stand back and review the purposes of reading. If we wish to read for pleasure, browse for interest or read an occasional article, then we can happily dip into whatever we choose, but, if we are making a determined effort to direct reading towards improving clinical care, then a more structured approach is needed. Our first goal must be to control what we read, and not let it control us.

The READER model (MacAuley, 1994) has been developed to help GPs approach reading in a structured way (see Fig. 14.1). It sets out some basic rules to help sort out what should be read. The criteria used are Relevance, Education, Applicability and Discrimination (quality of the methodology). The first principle is that we should select what to read by its relevance to our daily work, what changes we could make and if we can apply the lessons learned. Many factors determine if an article is relevant, but working in general practice we may choose to confine ourselves only to those articles that deal with general practice. The type of practice can be identified from the title, abstract and authors' qualifications, while a more detailed look at the article will give details about the circumstances, facilities and general background. If we cannot relate to the circumstances in which the research has been undertaken, it is doubtful if the article is relevant to us. Secondly, the article should tell us something new. If the general message is in keeping with what we already believe, then we are unlikely to change our behaviour, so perhaps the value of reading something that simply reinforces current practice should be questioned. These two criteria will filter out a lot of useless reading, but a third factor will help the selection. Even if an article is relevant to practice and could possibly lead to a change in our behaviour, it is of little value if we cannot carry this out in

Criteria	Possible score	Actual score
		(tick)
Relevance		
Not relevant to general practice	1	
Allied to general practice	2	
Only relevant to specialized general practice	3	
Broadly relevant to all general practice	4	
Relevant to me	5	
	Subtotal	
Education		
Would certainly not influence behaviour	1	
Could possibly influence behaviour	2	
Would cause reconsideration of behaviour	3	
Would probably alter behaviour	4	
Would definitely change behaviour	5	
	Subtotal	
Applicability		
Impossible in my practice	1	
Fundamental changes needed	2	
Perhaps possible	3	
Could be done with reorganization	4	
I could do that tomorrow	5	
	Subtotal	
Discrimination		
Poor descriptive study	1	
Moderately good descriptive study	2	
Good descriptive study but methods not reproducible	3	
Good descriptive study with sound methodology	4	
Single-blind study with attempts to control	5	
Controlled single-blind study	6	
Double-blind controlled study with method problem	7	
Double-blind controlled study with statistical deficiency	8	
Sound scientific paper with minor faults	9	
Scientifically sound paper	10	
	Subtotal	
	Total	

Figure 14.1 The READER method of critical reading.

our own practice. Thus the third criterion is that we should be able to apply the knowledge in practice. Armed with these three preliminary criteria, our reading can be greatly restricted. Certainly, something of value may be missed, but at least we can control what we can do, and banish the guilt that accompanies the pile of unread journals and magazines that we all have. Now that we are in charge of our reading, we can move on to look at the quality of what we read.

How to read and write

Until now we have concentrated on reading and in selecting what we should read. It is now appropriate to focus on the quality of the article. The qualities that are sought in reading are the same as those that should be included when writing. When the quality of an article is assessed, certain parameters should be focused on, and an author should address these same issues in a manuscript. The following sections describe the anatomy of a research article (MacAuley, 1995), and each component is as important for an aspiring author as it is to the reader in critical appraisal.

Abstract and introduction

A research article is usually written in a standard format with an Introduction, Methods, Results and Discussion (IMRAD). It is usually preceded by an abstract, and most high-quality journals use a structured abstract in the format Aims, Setting, Method, Results and Conclusion. The abstract should summarize the main findings and may act as a pointer to the quality of the study. It is important to study the abstract and, if writing, it is essential to get it right.

The introduction should set the scene. It should include a short review of the background to the study and discuss recent relevant work. This background indicates why the study was undertaken, clearly stating the aims and objectives of the work. It should be possible to jump directly to the discussion to see if these objectives have been achieved.

An investigator will usually have studied the literature before setting out on the study. In order to do this properly it is important to review the literature systematically. Using modern technology a very effective literature search can be undertaken and, although the methods are changing and evolving rapidly, recent guides are available (Greenhalgh, 1997a). Likewise, if reading an article, one should be happy that the author shows a good grasp of the relevant literature. In a review article, a systematic literature search is almost essential and a good review article will record the methods used to search and evaluate the relevant literature.

Methodology

When assessing the quality of a paper, the methods section is the most important. Methods lend credibility to the findings. The authors should explain what has been done, in sufficient detail for it to be reproduced by the reader. In some papers, the methods, questionnaires or tests may not be explained in detail, but they should be referenced so that the reader can retrieve them.

The authors should have made every effort to eliminate bias and Sackett and colleagues have noted 35 possible sources (Sackett, 1979). Sampling is a major possible source of bias in any study. The sampling method should be explicit and, in cross-sectional or descriptive studies, should be random, using mathematical formulae, random numbers or computer-generated random samples. Recruitment methods are another possible source of bias and they should be explicit. A particular problem can occur if there have been difficulties in recruiting participants and there has been a change in the recruitment methods or criteria during the study. The sample population determines how the results can be applied, so that if the sample is drawn from a particular subgroup, the results can only be applied to similar populations and cannot be generalized. For example, studies on hospital-based samples cannot always be applied to general-practice populations and vice versa. In case-control studies, the methods of selection of cases and controls should produce two groups that are as comparable as possible and the methods of selection and exclusion detailed to ensure that no unmatched factor could influence the result. As a minimum, the control group and cases should be matched for age and sex, but there are many other possible factors that can bias the results, depending on the type of study.

The randomized controlled trial (RCT) is an attempt to minimize sources of bias. The two groups of subjects are similar, and in the RCT the subjects are randomly allocated to intervention and control groups. If the trial is single-blind, then the investigator knows if subjects are in the intervention or control group, but, in a double-blind study, neither the investigator nor the subject knows which group they are in. The double-blind RCT is the gold standard or best available methodology. There are specific guidelines available for the publication of RCTs, and the CONSORT statement (Begg *et al.*, 1996), which sets standards for reporting such trials, includes a table and flow diagram, which are very useful to both reader and author.

The quality of the study is also determined by the quality of the measuring instrument. This could be a questionnaire, blood test or some other measurement. The quality or validity of this test has two dimensions: the accuracy of the test and its repeatability. Accuracy means that it measures specifically what it sets out to measure, but the accuracy of a measuring instrument may be refined even further into sensitivity and specificity. Sensitivity means that a test detects all those who have a certain characteristic and misses none, but may have some false positives. A very specific test detects only those who have a certain characteristic, but may miss some. These are false negatives.

Repeatability or reproducibility means that the test produces the same result when used on a number of occasions. Questionnaires should be validated and their repeatability demonstrated, or at least tested, in a pilot study. The repeatability values for blood tests should be given and the original work referenced. Similar criteria apply to other test instruments, such as sphygmomanometers, treadmills, etc.

Results and conclusions

Perhaps the most important component of the results is the response, as this indicates if the numbers included are adequate and representative. Even if all those who enter complete the study, it is only a small sample of the entire population and may not be representative. If only a small proportion of those who enter the study actually complete the study, then it is very unlikely to be representative. Response can be variable and influenced by many factors, but there may be some inherent factor in the study that influences response. In questionnaire studies every effort should be made to improve response, which usually includes at least two mailings and perhaps a telephone reminder. In such studies one aims for a 70% response, but in some general-practice studies the response may be as low as 25%. Poor response may also mask an inherent bias, so there should also be an effort to compare responders and non-responders, as there may be a differential response related to age, gender or perhaps smoking history, depending on the nature of the study.

In an intervention study, all those who enter the study should be accounted for. Those who do not complete the study cannot be ignored, because they may have dropped out for some reason related to the nature of the study. For example, they may suffer side effects, become ill or die or, in contrast, have such an improvement that they do not feel the need to return to follow up. Those who do not complete the study may have had a profound effect on the result had they been included, so they cannot be ignored.

A result may be inconclusive for other reasons. If the sample size is too small or the numbers in each subgroup are insufficient to show a statistically significant difference, then the study may produce a false-negative result even when there are real differences. Such a false-negative result is known as a type II error. The ability to demonstrate statistical differences is the power of a study, and is a mathematical function of the number of participants, so it should be possible to calculate the power of a study in advance. In contrast, small differences between groups can be statistically significant in very large studies, so the result may be significant but mean little. Confounding factors, which affect both the subject of the study and the population, may affect the results, and the most common confounding factors include age, body mass and smoking.

Readers and authors should pay particular attention to illustrations and graphs. While an illustration may take the place of much explanation, it is also possible to mislead by changing the emphasis of the results. This may result from modification of the units, spacing or axis of the graph.

Statistics often frighten GPs. They are, however, simply a measure of chance. In any study, there is a possibility that a positive result could have occurred by chance and statistics are a mathematical method of estimating this likelihood. By convention, if we believe there is a less than 1 in 20 chance that the result was a fluke, we accept the result. In this case the P (probability) value is less than 0.05 ($P < 0.05$). Confidence intervals are now used more commonly, as they offer a range of values within which a true result is likely to occur. With 95% confidence intervals, there is a 95% likelihood that the true value is within this range.

Statistical significance and clinical significance are two common terms used in medical literature. Statistical significance is simply a mathematical means of estimating if a result could have occurred by chance. It means nothing to patient care, medical management or treatment; it is just a mathematical formula. Statistical tests are used as a convenient means of deciding if a result should be believed. What these results mean in medical management is a different issue and clinical significance is the term that helps us to interpret findings. In reading or writing research, the reader and author should address both these issues. Firstly, is the result statistically significant, if we believe it, and, secondly, if we believe the result, what should it mean to medical management? When a decision is made about an individual patient at a particular time in a particular context, the research results are interpreted using an additional factor—personal significance (Sweeney *et al.*, 1998).

The discussion section of the paper should review the results in context, explore possible errors, recognize misinterpretations and draw a balanced conclusion. The interpretation should match the results and the conclusions not exaggerate the findings. The results should be reviewed in the context of recent literature and clinical management and the authors may highlight strengths and weaknesses of their own work.

There is a hierarchy in design. Case-studies are the weakest form of evidence, because they may represent an isolated finding which cannot be generalized. Observational studies demonstrate a cross-sectional effect, but evidence is stronger than in a case-control study. A cohort study shows changes over time, while a double-blind RCT is the highest-quality methodology available in medical research. The READER model recognizes this hierarchy and applies a score to each methodology (see Fig. 14.1).

Other methods

Not everyone is comfortable with epidemiological concepts and the rules used to measure the validity of research. Some are put off by the detail required or the apparent skills necessary to undertake critical appraisal. There are short cuts. Most articles in high-quality journals are peer-reviewed, so that articles published in these journals have usually been critically appraised by two or more experts in the field. They will already have assessed the quality of the article on your behalf and the editor will have taken the decision on publication based on their opinion. The more respected and well known the journal, the lower the proportion of submitted articles that are published and, as a result, the quality should be higher. One may depend on the reviewers and assume that articles published in a particular journal are of good quality. This is a reasonably safe strategy, but, even if the quality of the articles is good, the content may not be of interest or relevant to you, so you may have to look elsewhere if searching for a particular subject.

One way to keep up to date is to decide to read only review articles. By restricting yourself to review articles in a respected journal, the quality can be reasonably assured, but the content cannot be chosen. There can be a variable quality in review articles too, which has led to a further set of ground rules for the appraisal of review articles (Greenhalgh, 1997b). Review articles should be written in a structured manner and, just as in original research, the methods section is the most important. The authors should make explicit how they searched out the papers used in referencing the review and what criteria were used in assessing the quality of these papers. Unless the review has been approached in an objective structured format, then the article is simply an opinion.

A further approach is a journal club. This format has now evolved from informal meetings to more structured group sessions in critical appraisal. The journal club offers a useful opportunity for assessing articles, and is a valuable educational exercise in its own right (Linzer, 1987). Any individual can study the methods used in critical appraisal, but the journal club provides the opportunity to learn from others. It has been used as an educational exercise in teaching critical reading in a postgraduate setting (Alguire *et al.*, 1988; Konen & Fromm, 1990), and interest in participation in a journal club has been shown to relate to ability to criticize the literature (Heligman, 1991). An interesting feature is that participants' opinion of the quality of the medical literature may be lower after learning about critical appraisal, and some have been so disillusioned that they questioned the value of continuing to read. Most journal clubs appraise two journals in 1 hour, usually during lunchtime, and high attendance rates are associated with high-quality academic leadership (Sidorov, 1995).

A further variation of the journal club is the clinical debate, first described in 1982 (Woods & Winkel, 1982). In the traditional journal club, participants either review a single article, read the classic articles or learn about experimental design. This further variation is based on 'creating a controversy' and has now evolved into the debate format. One problem is that the subject chosen must be controversial (Douglas, 1994), so offering two sides to the argument, which limits the potential subject matter. It also demands a lot of work by the moderator (Abyad, 1995).

There has been little published research on the effectiveness of teaching critical appraisal, although empirically we believe it to be useful. There is some evidence that teaching critical appraisal can improve knowledge, but there is no evidence to demonstrate that it can change behaviour. In one study of residents, there was a statistically significant improvement in knowledge (21% of the intervention residents improved their test scores by $\geq$ 18% compared with control residents) after their intervention (Kitchens & Pfeifer, 1989). In a similar study among medical students, knowledge could similarly be improved (Bennett *et al.*, 1987) (40% of the intervention group improved their knowledge compared with 13 controls). Sackett (1990), the doyen of critical appraisal, put these achievements in perspective, using the 'number needed to treat' as a model, and demonstrated that, using this method of teaching, all residents would improve their knowledge in 48 weeks and the medical students in 32 weeks. The key issue is whether learning the skills of critical reading can change behaviour. For all the discussion about the benefits of critical reading and learning the skills of critical reading, there is little evidence that reading influences what doctors do and the outcome for patients.

So you have decided to write!

Those in academic departments and research practices are expected to publish, but other GPs may have carried out an interesting study or made an unusual observation and wish to bring it to the attention of a wider audience. Getting published for the first time is challenging, and it may be easiest to begin with a case report or letter to the editor. To publish a more substantial paper requires considerable thought and planning. The guidelines for reading and writing given in this chapter may help, but it is always useful to seek advice from someone with knowledge and experience in publication before submission. The peer-review system can be quite intimidating for aspiring authors. Submitting your piece of research to critical appraisal can sometimes be bruising, but remember that it is rare to get a glowing review and the review, however harsh, will always be of help in rewriting a paper for resubmission elsewhere. Look upon it as a learning experience. If your paper is accepted, it is a triumph, but if it is rejected, look at it again and if, on second thoughts, you agree with the referee then bin it. If you can rewrite and improve it, then there are many more journals!

Conclusion

Reading medical literature and assessing the quality of research are among the cornerstones of evidence-based medicine. As evidence-based medicine begins to change the nature of decision making in clinical care, including general practice, the skills of reading and writing are likely to become increasingly important. GPs are now more aware of the need to justify clinical decisions with evidence, but seeking out and assessing the quality of evidence in the literature is a relatively new skill. This chapter illustrates some of the criteria used in deciding what to read and the parameters to be examined in an appraisal.

The qualities that we seek in reading research evidence are the very same qualities that we must include when writing a manuscript. Evidence-based medicine in primary care should be driven by evidence from research undertaken in primary care. But general practice, and the academic community in particular, are beginning to realize that there has been relatively little research from general practice to drive the decision-making process. Hence the increased investment in and expansion of academic general practice and NHS research and development focus on primary care. Research undertaken will be written up, but the quality of writing will determine if it is published and how it is appraised and interpreted.

General practice is both an art and a science. We all have a responsibility to integrate the science into daily practice, but we can only discover the science through our reading, and can only expand our scientific knowledge through research and publication. Just as research and clinical care weave the pattern of patient management in general practice, so critical appraisal of the literature (reading) and the ability to compose a research paper (writing) are two complementary skills woven together.

References

Abyad, A. (1995) Debate journal club teaches critical appraisal skills. *Family Medicine* **27**, 226–227.

Alguire, P.C., Massa, M.D., Lienhart, K.W. & Henry, R.C. (1988) A packaged workshop for teaching critical reading of the medical literature. *Medical Teacher* **10**, 85–90.

Begg, C., Cho, M., Eastwood, S. *et al.* (1996) Improving the quality of reporting of randomised controlled trials. The CONSORT statement. *Journal of the American Medical Association* **276**, 637–639.

Bennett, K.J., Sackett, D.L., Haynes, R.B., Neufield, V.R., Tugwell, P. & Roberts, R. (1987) A controlled trial of teaching critical appraisal of the clinical literature to medical students. *Journal of the American Medical Association* **257**, 2451–2454.

Covell, D.G., Uman, G.C. & Manning, P.R. (1985) Information needs in office practice: are they being met? *Annals of Internal Medicine* **103**, 596–599.

Curry, L. & Putnam, R.W. (1981) Continuing medical education in maritime Canada; the methods physicians use, would prefer and find most effective. *Canadian Medical Association Journal* **124**, 563–566.

Douglas, M. (1994) Use of the debate format journal club to teach critical appraisal. *Family Medicine* **27**, 414.

Greenhalgh, T. (ed.) (1997a) Searching the literature. In: *How to Read a Paper—The Basics of Evidence Based Medicine*, pp. 13–30. BMJ Publishing Group, London.

Greenhalgh, T. (ed.) (1997b) Papers that summarise other papers (systematic reviews and meta-analyses). In: *How to Read a Paper—The Basics of Evidence Based Medicine*, pp. 111–128. BMJ Publishing Group, London.

Heligman, R.M. (1991) Resident evaluation of a family practice residency journal club. *Family Medicine* **23**, 152–153.

Jones, R. (1991) Critical reading [editorial]. *Family Practice* **8**, 1–2.

Kitchens, J.M. & Pfeifer, M.P. (1989) Teaching residents to read the medical literature: a controlled trial of a curriculum in critical appraisal/clinical epidemiology. *Journal of General Internal Medicine* **4**, 384–387.

Konen, J.C. & Fromm, B.S. (1990) A family practice residency curriculum in critical appraisal of the medical literature. *Family Medicine* **22**, 284–287.

Linzer, M. (1987) The journal club and medical education: over 100 years of unrecorded history. *Postgraduate Medical Journal* **63**, 475–478.

MacAuley, D. (1994) READER: an acronym to aid critical reading in general practice. *British Journal of General Practice* **44**, 83–85.

MacAuley, D. (1995) Critical appraisal of medical literature: an aid to rational decision making. *Family Medicine* **12**, 98–103.

Sackett, D.L. (1979) Bias in analytic research. *Journal of Chronic Disease* **32**, 51–63.

Sackett, D.L. (1990) Teaching critical appraisal [letter]. *Journal of General Internal Medicine* **5**, 272.

Sidorov, J. (1995) How are internal medicine residency journal clubs organised and what makes them successful? *Archives of Internal Medicine* **155**, 1193–1197.

Smith, R. (1996) What clinical information do doctors need? *British Medical Journal* **313**, 1062.

Stinson, E.R. & Mueller, D.A. (1980) Survey of health professional information habits and needs conducted through personal experience. *Journal of the American Medical Association* **243**, 140–143.

Sweeney, K., MacAuley, D.C. & Pereira Gray, D.J. (1998) Personal significance; the third dimension. *Lancet* **351**, 134–136.

Woods, J.R. & Winkel, C.E. (1982) Journal club format emphasising techniques for critical reading. *Journal of Medical Education* **57**, 799–801.

15 Practice systems

The theory: improving practice systems

Running a practice is the art of modelling systems we do not wholly understand into activities we cannot precisely analyse so as to cope with demands we cannot properly assess in such a way that no one suspects the extent of our ignorance.

What are we trying to achieve in this chapter?

The aims of this chapter can be summarized as:
- To help you change your practice systems to provide higher quality care at lower cost.
- To encourage the use of continuing quality improvement methods to change your practice systems.
- To ask and answer five important questions about change and improvement in practice systems:
    - I What are you trying to achieve?
    - II What do you either know or need to know about this subject to plan change?
    - III How will you know if the proposed change is an improvement?
    - IV What changes can you make?
    - V How will you continue the improvement in a cycle of feedback and change?

What do you either know or need to know about this subject to plan change?

Why try to provide higher quality care at lower cost?
We are searching for the holy grail of health care.

Governments strive to purchase and provide better national health-care systems. The current optimal model is a 'lean system'. This jargon is borrowed from the car industry, which had three main stages in the last century. The first stage was when craftsmen specially made each car. 'Craft production' provided high-quality cars at high prices, but these were too expensive for most people. Next came Henry Ford's innovative 'mass production' that made cheaper cars of lower quality available to the masses. Quality has improved in the last 20 years, with Japanese-type 'lean production' that makes high-quality cars at low cost. These three production concepts can be used to describe medical practice today. All systems are unsatisfactory. In the USA the rising costs of 'craft care' may become too expensive to be affordable, and in the UK the quality of 'mass care' (especially the long delays for patients to see specialists) is a constant source of irritation to everyone. The new approach in the world health-care systems is to provide both higher quality and lower cost—an evidence-based, managed-care or lean-medicine system.

Modern general-practice systems are expected to provide high-quality low-cost care, and continuous quality improvement methods seem the best way to achieve this goal.

What is high quality and low cost?

It depends where you start.

You can represent different aspects of quality by the six sides of a cube (see Fig. 15.1) and assess the different aspects of quality you provide by asking these six questions about the quality of your service:

1 Access: Is there access to care or are there barriers to the service? For example, how long does it take for a patient to get an appointment with the doctor?

2 Best treatments: Are the best, most effective, treatments available? For example, does the doctor recommend evidence-based treatments?

3 Customer satisfaction: Are the customers satisfied and pleased with the service they receive? For example, would they recommend their doctor to their friends?

4 Depth of care: Is there a depth of care, with the wider issues of public health addressed? For example, are 'at-risk' patients,

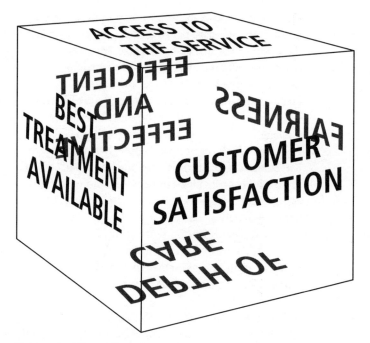

Figure 15.1 The quality cube.

such as asplenic patients, searched for and offered pneumococcal immunization?

5 Efficiency and effectiveness: Is the care provided efficient and effective, with value for money? For example, are the rates of investigation, prescription and referral appropriate?

6 Fairness: Is the care fairly available, with the opportunities the same for all patients and groups? For example, are the elderly housebound diabetics offered the same standard of care as those who are ambulatory?

Quality can only be achieved by addressing all six sides of the cube. For instance, do you provide a high-quality service if you always give the best treatments but your patients have to wait a month to see you?

What are your standards for quality and cost?

If you do not know what you are trying to do, how will you know when you've done it?

Quality standards can be minimal, optimal or ideal. The minimum is the standard below which performance is unacceptable, the optimum is the best attainable with available resources and conditions, and the ideal is the best that could be achieved if there were no constraints. National quality schemes set the optimal quality standards for practice systems. In the UK, quality standards are set by schemes like the Fellowship by Assessment of the Royal College of General Practitioners (RCGP), the RCGP Quality Practice Award, Investors in People, British Standard BS5750, the King's Fund Quality Initiative and the Charter Mark. None of these schemes provides standards for all aspects of quality, but each can provide a challenge for a practice trying to attain a higher standard of performance.

Cost standards can be derived from your practice's historical costs or comparative national figures (in the UK, they are published in monthly magazines such as *Medeconomics* and *Financial Pulse*). These set standards for your present or future performance.

Why are change and improvement necessary?
> If you do it the way you've always done it, you'll get what you always had!

The aim is to decide which changes will make your practice high-quality and low-cost that will hopefully also make the practice systems better and easier to operate. The usual questions a new GP asks are:

- How does the system work?
- Why does it work like this?
- Does it need changing?

Every practice has a history of change, and you should try to discover how and why the present practice systems have evolved. If you want to understand your practice's systems, you must also understand how to make changes and improvements in your practice. Most GPs are not trained to fix things that are not broken and so you may only notice a practice system when there is a problem. Even in the best practices things do go wrong. When change is inevitable, some improvement is usually possible. GPs have different ways of approaching problems, and business-management books promote different approaches. All these approaches to improving practice systems are based on our different assumptions or prejudices about human behaviour and change. This chapter gives a simple, continuous, quality-improvement approach to looking at practice systems that you can adapt to your own preferred style.

What is continuous quality improvement?

> Improvement is no accident. It requires aim. Implementing change and improvement is usually not a single action but involves a well planned stepwise process including a combination of interventions linked to specific obstacles to change. All the different approaches for changing clinical practice may be valuable and effective provided they are adapted to the specific feature of the change proposed, the target group, the setting and the obstacles to change encountered. (Grol, 1997)

If you do want to improve your practice you need to understand 'improvement knowledge'.

Batalden and Stoltz (1993) produced a framework for the continual improvement of health care, and this is detailed below.

Knowledge. Professional knowledge and improvement knowledge are needed:

1 Your professional knowledge: for instance, if you are trying to improve your prescribing you have your professional knowledge on the:
- Subject—for example, pharmacology.
- Discipline—for example, family practice.
- Values—for example, sharing the clinical decision making with your patients, the purchasers and other providers of care.

2 Your improvement knowledge: you also need knowledge about how systems work. This includes the:
- Variation in systems—common causes, special causes and tampering (see below).
- Psychology of team working—people are the single most important asset. People make things happen, they get the results.
- Theory of knowledge—theory needs to be linked to practice. Planning is not enough, projects need to get into action.

It is only through mistakes that learning and change can happen. Trying things out in audit Plan/Do/Study/Act (PDSA) cycles should become a normal way of running a practice.

Leadership. Leaders need to have:
- Vision—a clear understanding of the purpose of the practice.
- Visibility—be accountable for their actions. They should follow the plan only as long as it gets results and continue change only until the aims are achieved.
- Value—with sufficient expertise and empathy to integrate the leadership policies with the practice's commonly shared values.

Tools and method. There are a collection of tried and tested tools that can help the improvement process, such as:
- Process system—a system map like a flowchart.
- Group process and collaborative work—facilitate working with others; for example, brainstorming, rank ordering.
- Statistical thinking—for example, run charts, scatter diagrams.
- Planning and analysis—for example, allow processing of qualitative data.

Daily work applications. You need:
- Models for testing change and making improvement—removing the special causes of variation to improve stability and predictability (see below).
- Reviews of improvement—systematic enquiry to promote learning and accelerate improvement.

Why does performance vary in a stable practice system?
> Every system is perfectly designed to achieve the results it gets.

Variations are the point-to-point differences in performance of a system measured over time. They are always present in systems. The founder of modern quality control was Walter Shewhart, who worked at the Bell Laboratories in the USA in the 1920s and developed insights into the nature of variation in manufacturing and ways to minimize it. His work was first published in his book *Economic Control of Quality of Manufactured Product* in 1931.

His associate W. Edwards Deming edited Shewhart's second book, *Statistical Methods from the Viewpoint of Quality Control* (Shewhart, 1939). Deming went on, over the next 60 years, to extend the paradigm to other commercial activities and played a major role in developing modern Japanese manufacturing techniques. One of the major contributions he made was to understand why performance varies in stable systems. A stable practice system is one in which the way of working has settled down into a well-used and familiar pattern. As an example, most GPs will be familiar with the traditional handwritten paper medical record. Before it was replaced with the computerized electronic health record (EHR), it was a familiar and stable system. Shewhart and Deming showed that the performance in any stable system is a characteristic of the system. In this example, the handwritten paper medical records in general practice were associated with performance problems like 'lost' notes, illegible handwriting and difficulty in finding the important bit of information when required. Only changes in the system, not adjustments to the existing way of working (which is already stable), can lessen the variation in system performance. This defect rate (e.g. the common occurrence of lost notes) is a property of the system and to reduce the defect rate the system must be improved.

Not all changes will make things better. The only way of being certain is to try it on a small scale. Before the use of computer systems, practices tried all sorts of changes to try to improve paper notes. An alternative system to handwritten paper medical records is the EHR. The EHR can solve problems like illegible handwriting, missing records and relational databases, but it has different performance characteristics, for instance it does not work without electricity.

There are two main ways of acting on a stable system, either by change leading to improvement or by change making things worse. Change without a systematic approach to improvement is more likely to make the system worse.

What are the common mistakes?
The following common mistakes can be made:
1 You try to fix something which is not broken! You mistake the cause of the variation as being special in nature, when in fact it is

random and caused by the system (this is known as a common cause of variation). For example, when we used paper medical records in the practice, we would sometimes lose notes. The reception staff knew where to look for most lost notes and the notes would eventually be found. This regular loss of notes is a common cause of variation and can occur in unusual ways. The notes of one patient were lost and seemed impossible to find. All the doctors denied responsibility, until the following winter when one of the doctors put on the winter coat he used for visiting patients at home and discovered the missing notes in the pocket! Although this seems extraordinary, this is simply a common cause of variation inherent in having paper medical records. The notes can be misplaced in many different ways and you can take no sensible action to stop it recurring.

2 You do not recognize a fault when you see it. You mistake the source of the variation as being a common cause, when in fact it is special in nature (this is known as a special cause) and can and should be identified and, if possible, eliminated. Paper medical records were lost because one doctor would take the records home to write medical reports and the notes would get left at home. This is a special cause; it can be identified and action (such as preventing the forgetful doctor from taking records home) should be taken to stop it recurring.

3 You tamper with the system. You make overadjustments or react inappropriately to the variation in performance. It usually makes things worse. It happens when the problem in a system is misunderstood and attempts to fix a problem are misdirected. An example of tampering could be locking up the patients' paper medical records in the belief that this will reduce the number of lost notes.

4 You prioritize the wrong changes. The aim is to understand what tasks you need to do and in what order. Important but non-urgent business (like planning a switch from paper records to EHRs) should take priority over urgent but non-important interruptions (like most telephone calls).

5 You become more concerned with process than outcome. The ultimate purpose of practice systems is to improve the outcome, not the process. Most successful organizations set managers clear goals and give them autonomy to reach them in their own way.

For example, your main concern should be that the patients' notes are available when you (or others) need them.

6 You focus on databases rather than data uses. All the data you collect must have a purpose. Collection without use is pointless. Data are useful for the assessment of achievement (what you have done), aptitude (what you should be able to do), competence (what you can do) and performance (what you really do). A commitment to regular assessment of your practice's systems, with a cycle of follow-up to overcome any constraints to learning, change and improvement, mimics the audit cycle.

Is there an alternative viewpoint?

There are two possible ways for us to proceed. One is the automated, mechanistic, defined way and the other is the soft, instinctive, natural way. The first can't cope with the complexity of life and provides no reason for living; the second leaves mankind blind, lacking in plan and vulnerable to all sorts of dangers. (Willis, 1995)

The view is that rule makers or practice-system designers can never describe life, they can only set the limits. The common sense of people must be used to balance the forces for change, quality improvement and technological progress. These two views are not incompatible, in that rules can be made to be flexible and common sense can become more informed common sense.

How will you know if the changes are an improvement?

You must decide on your success criteria before you start; they will be related to your original aims.

What changes can you make?

Build improvement into your changes

Before you change your system, you must understand your aims. There are five questions worth asking whenever **any** change is suggested:

   I What are you trying to achieve?
   II What do you either know or need to about this subject to plan change?

III How will you know if the proposed change is an improvement?

IV What changes can you make?

V How will you continue improvement in a cycle of feedback and change?

What should you do first?

Don't try to sell elastic by the metre!

Your performance will be limited by your competence, motivation and resources. Lack of performance may be due to a specific block or constraint. All your systems cannot be improved at once, so you should learn to prioritize your efforts (by understanding your motivation) and increase your competence (by understanding improvement theory).

Motivation. This occurs when you discover a perception of need that creates an anxiety that compels you to act. The need is the discrepancy between what is and what ought to be. Customary gaps are the small discrepancies between what is and what ought to be. These small gaps have little effect on motivation. Very large gaps block change, because they produce high levels of anxiety and cause aversion, rather than reducing need. You should target your changes on gaps in your performance that are achievable.

Competence. Make an honest assessment of your current competence and what you can do to improve it.

Resources. These include the existing practice structure, protected time and support from the purchasers, other providers and your patients. For instance, if you are adequately resourced for a difficult change, then high performance is possible, but, if you are poorly resourced, you will be more at risk of personal stress and burn-out.

What are the common areas for improvement?

Berwick (1994) has suggested some priorities for improvement in health care. These include:

• Reduce waiting times: Decrease patients' waiting in all its forms. Ask when the service is needed and match the supply to the demand.

- Reduce wasteful and duplicative recording: Reduce the frequency of duplicate data entry and of recording of information never used. Doctors, nurses and reception staff often record the same information on different systems. The burden of work is made worse when paper records are maintained in addition to new computer recording. Use data rather than collect data.
- Increase the appropriateness of care and stop procedures that do not help: All practices have a legacy of unnecessary procedures. You should identify these and stop them!
- Increase effective preventive practices.
- Rationalize pharmaceutical use.
- Involve patients in decisions: Try to increase the patients' active participation in decision making about the clinical options. You can increase quality of care and costs can go down, because patients do not always choose expensive care.

How will you continue improvement in a cycle of feedback and change?

> I am not certain when I first realized that it would never be possible for me to understand the system of quality improvement 'all at once'. But that thought, when it did come, was actually a relief. It was both challenging and invigorating to grasp that the general issues of improvement in complex, human systems are far too ranging, too interactive and too interesting for one to grip as if they were a hammer. (Berwick, 1993)

You should:
- Decide on your priorities.
- Compare your practice's performance against internal and/or external standards.
- Question your practice systems' performances.
- Understand the limitations of your systems—differentiate between the causes that can be corrected and the inherent limitations.
- Decide if your practice systems can be improved.
- Consider new practice systems to service existing or new areas of concern.
- Build teams to help you—you need a practice team that is an asset rather than just a cost.

- Use these continuous quality-improvement methods to guide changes.

An example: improving the practice's appointments systems

This example of the application of continuous quality improvement is based on an article first published in *Financial Pulse* (Kemple, 1997).

There is a myth that you increase patient demand by providing more appointments and you can limit patient demand by reducing appointments. In fact, this is an example of a stable practice system where there is a finite number of patients who are ever likely to need or want to see you in a day. Tampering with the system can make patients and practices groan with the pressure of demand. The gap between what most patients want (an appointment with the doctor of their choice at a time of their choice) and what most GPs can provide (either an appointment with the duty doctor on the same day or an appointment with the doctor of the patient's choice some time later) will continue, unless there is a change. Examples of this change could be a huge expansion in primary care or a major system change in the way that primary care is delivered.

The challenge is to accept your patients' expectations and demands for appointments and try to improve the way you manage demands for appointments.

What are you trying to achieve?

Expectations vary between practices, but you can decide what you think you should achieve. The RCGP's Fellowship by Assessment (Version 9 in 1998/99, Royal College of General Practitioners, 1996) has suggested the following criteria, to which you can add your own standards:

- The doctor is available at specified times for surgery consultations and telephone advice.
- The system for monitoring appointments is capable of identifying and correcting significant delays, irrespective of the type of appointment system, if any, that is employed.

- For urgent matters, the patient is able to see his or her own doctor or partner or deputy at the next surgery, or speak with the duty doctor.
- For routine matters, the patient is usually offered the opportunity to see the doctor of his or her own choice within a period set by the practice and published to the patients.

What do you either know or need to know about this subject to plan change?

What is the best way to manage appointments?
There is no clear answer. Audits of appointments systems have proliferated, but at the time of writing (1998) these, and the rest of the GP literature, had not provided the answers. All the published work antedates the computerized appointment systems which have changed many practices' paper systems.

How many appointments do you need to supply each week to match the normal demands?
Each week there is a minimum number of appointments that will always be necessary. If you provide less than your minimum number of appointments, you will put yourself under extra pressure, and cause general dissatisfaction to patients, staff and doctors.

Your own past performance will give you an answer. Your computer or your appointments book should provide the total number of patients seen in the past year. Divide this total by 52 and you have a number that you can use as your starting-point for deciding how many appointments you need to provide each week to meet the normal demands. You may need to supply 5–10% less appointments in predictably quiet times (such as the summer) or 5–10% more at busy times (such as the winter).

How do you iron out the peaks and troughs in demand for appointments?
Peaks and troughs are usually daily or weekly. If you provide appointments throughout the working day rather than have all doctors consulting at the same fixed times in morning and evening surgeries, there will be a less stressful and more consistent flow

of work through the day. The weekly peaks and troughs are either predictable or unpredictable and either true or false. Some of the causes of these peaks and troughs are described below:

- Predictable and true variations can happen with seasonal changes, such as flu-vaccination campaigns and patients' summer holidays.
- Predictable and false variations may be a result of the loss of appointments at Bank Holidays, so that 5 days' demand must be satisfied in 4 days.
- Unpredictable and false variations are caused by changes in the number of doctors supplying appointments rather than the number of patients demanding appointments. If too many doctors are absent, the remaining doctors will experience a peak in the demand for appointments.
- Unpredictable and true peaks and troughs happen with the excess demand in flu epidemics and a sudden drop in demand in snowstorms.

You can identify and correct all the peaks and troughs in advance, except the truly unpredictable ones.

Will the other doctors want to change?

Traditionally, many GPs find the concept of customer service difficult and this makes satisfying patients' expectations more challenging. How many GPs with school-age children will respond with enthusiasm to the need to reduce their own holiday entitlements to provide the required number of appointments during the school holidays? Active planning to employ extra deputy doctors during school holidays may be the only answer.

How do you allow for the differing consulting styles of your partners?

First, be sure you know what you are trying to achieve. For example your problem may be that one partner consults more slowly than the others and cannot keep up with the usual pace of the practice. This problem could be tackled by encouraging personal responsibility in partners by having personal lists. If you publish each partner's personal standards for availability and care, patients can make an informed choice about whom they want to have as their personal doctor and accept the differing consulting styles. It may be that the slower doctor is a popular doctor. If the slower doctor is also an unpopular doctor, you may have a problem partner! This is a special cause of variation!

How should you deal with non-urgent appointments?
If you have supplied enough 'urgent' appointments, patients can be directed for follow-up or for routine matters to see the doctor of their own choice within a period set by the practice and published to the patients. Many GPs work part-time and so they will never be available on a daily basis for their patients. If you tell patients what to expect, then they can decide if they want to switch to another doctor who is available sooner or wait more than a few days to see the doctor they know. If your patients start to desert you, then you will know you will have either to improve upon the standard you provide for your existing patients or to practise with a smaller list size!

How will you know if the proposed change is an improvement?

You must decide how you will measure your success. This might be:
- Using locums less (or more).
- Having less 'urgent' patients squeezed into or at the end of surgery time.
- Having greater continuity of care.
- Improving measured patient satisfaction.
- Fewer complaints.
- Reducing the number of days' wait for a non-urgent appointment.
- Less waiting for an urgent appointment.
- More telephone appointments.
- Lower patient waiting times.
- Fewer patients who do not attend for their booked appointments.
- A shift in your workload from home visits to surgery appointments to telephone appointments or other contacts.

What changes can you make?

This will vary from practice to practice. A common problem is likely to be trying to match patients' requests for appointment times with the doctor of their choice in the next few days. Some strategies include making the practice's 'duty doctor' provide only quick or urgent appointments, rather like the fast queue at supermarket tills; others involve making doctors' appointments available sequentially, so that some of the consultations cannot be booked more that 24–48 hours in advance, or scheduling telephone appointments.

Another common problem is that too many doctors are absent from the practice at the same time. Discipline is needed to stop this, by enforcing a strict rule about how many doctors can be absent at the same time, but it helps to avoid the undersupply of appointments.

How will you continue improvement in a cycle of feedback and change?

Once you use the simple five-question checklist, it is easy to repeat the process:

I   What are you trying to achieve?
II What do you either know or need to know about this subject to plan change?
III How will you know if the proposed change is an improvement?
IV What changes can you make?
V   How will you continue improvement in a cycle of feedback and change?

Decide if your outcome measures have been achieved, review the whole process, and then make your next improvement in your practice's systems.

References

Batalden, P. & Stoltz, P. (1993) A framework for continual improvement of health care. *The Joint Commission Journal on Quality Improvement* **19**, 424–447.

Berwick, D. (1993) Eleven worthy aims for clinical leadership of Health System Reform. *Joint Commission Journal on Quality Improvement* **19**, 449–456.

Grol, R. (1997) Beliefs and evidence in changing clinical practice. *British Medical Journal* **315**, 418–421.

Kemple, T. (1997) Educate your patients to reduce demand. *Financial Pulse* **12**, 38–44.

Royal College of General Practitioners (1998) *Fellowship by Assessment.* Criteria and User's Guide, 9th Version. RCGP, London.

Royal College of General Practitioners (1997) *Quality Practice Award, Version 2.* RCGP, North East Scotland Faculty.

Shewhart, W. (1931) *Economic Control of Quality of Manufactured Product.* Van Nostrand Co. Inc., New York.

Shewhart, W. (1939) *Statistical Methods from the Viewpoint of Quality Control* (ed. W.E. Deming). The Graduate School, Washington.

Willis, J. (1995) *The Paradox of Progress.* Radcliffe Medical Press, Oxford.

Further reading

Baron, R. & Greenberg, J. (1990) *Behavior in Organizations: Understanding and Managing the Human Side of Work.* Allyn and Bacon, London.

Brooks, J. & Borgardts, I. (1994) *Total Quality in General Practice.* Radcliffe Medical Press, Oxford.

Senge, P. (1992) *The Fifth Discipline: The Art and Practice of the Learning Organization.* Century Business, London.

16   Continuing your education

The registrar year is over. Summative assessment has been negotiated and passed. It's time perhaps to throw away the video camera, to put the textbooks back on the library shelf and to leave audit to the enthusiasts. This is an understandable enough feeling, but by the time you have finished reading this chapter I hope you will agree with me that further education is useful, indeed essential, and that it can be fun.

The sections of this chapter are:
- Why continuing education?
- Principles of adult learning.
- Opportunities for education.
- The practice as a learning environment.
- Accreditation of education.
- Fellowship of the RCGP by assessment.

The intention is first to help you understand why it is worth bothering with further education. This will be reinforced by a discussion of the principles of learning and how education can be useful, supportive and fun. There will then be an attempt to outline the types of educational opportunity that are available. Details of courses, etc., change all the time so it would be inappropriate to give a detailed guide, rather a pointer to what to look for and where to look. This is the longest section of the chapter, ranging over traditional methods of continuing education to more appropriate ways of developing professionally. There then follows a short section on learning within the practice, its advantages and disadvantages and how to go about it. Then a section (which, in 1999, may have to be to some extent speculative) on how your education might be accredited follows. Such accreditation is currently important financially and it may, in the future, be essential for continued permission to practise. Finally, Fellowship by Assessment is mentioned briefly, as this incorporates so many good ideas on education and accreditation.

Why continuing education?

I completed my vocational training in 1974. Just consider a few of the changes related to general practice (and also included are a few points on the history of GP education) that have happened since then:

- Crucial therapeutic advances, such as antiulcer drugs, ACE inhibitors and calcium channel blockers.
- Huge advances in surgery, such as the development of 'keyhole' surgery, leading to vastly shorter stays in hospital.
- The NHS has been reorganized countless times. None of the health authorities that existed in 1974 (at least in England and Wales) exist now, the internal market has come and (probably) gone, GP fundholding has come and is going ... the list is endless.
- Primary health-care teams were extremely rudimentary in 1974. Even my training practice, a leading 'academic' practice, did not have a practice nurse and 'attached staff' were a novelty.
- In 1974, vocational training for general practice was voluntary and many districts had not yet established training schemes. While going into general practice straight from preregistration posts was becoming less common, few doctors undertook a full 3 years of vocational training.
- Only a handful of medical schools had a professor of general practice in 1974. Now all UK schools do, and some have more than one.
- Until 1990, GPs were reimbursed under Section 63 for the expenses of their education at approved courses. In 1974, such courses were fairly few and far between, with hospital postgraduate centres just beginning to become established.

Without labouring the point any further, it must be obvious that GPs have had to adapt to these changes and countless others. If there is one certainty about the future, it is that changes will continue and that the rate of change may well continue to increase. Perhaps the main purpose of continuing education (or continuing professional development, as it is probably more appropriately called) is to help GPs to anticipate these changes and cope with them. Professional fulfilment will be even greater if doctors can play a part in instigating changes and not just react to them. There is clearly much more to continuing education than just 'keeping up to date', important as that is.

In today's rapidly changing world, GP principals remain (but possibly not for much longer) in an unusual position. They have almost complete job security but they have very little chance of career development. Once you are a partner on parity, you may stay in the same job all your working life with no chance of 'promotion'. Therefore much of the professional development that would have been provided as a matter of course in other professions has to be worked at if burn-out is to be avoided. Your continuing education needs to consider yourself as a person and how you are going to develop and continue to find the job fulfilling. Many GPs find that it helps to engage in 'outside' medical activities, which, as well as being interesting and sometimes financially rewarding, can add a stimulus to day-to-day work in the surgery. Planning these activities is another important part of professional development.

So continuing professional development is important for:
- Coping with change.
- Enhancing your career.
- Preventing burn-out.
- Keeping up to date.
- Making the job more interesting.
- (Before too long) continued permission to practise.
  Welcome on board!

Principles of adult learning

The essential theory of adult learning has been encapsulated in an ancient Chinese proverb:
> I hear and I forget
> I see and I remember
> I do and I understand

This simply means that the more we are involved in the learning experience, the more we are likely to benefit from it. There is ample evidence of the truth of this assertion, even for those of us whose learning style (see Chapter 4) is more towards the 'theorist' end of the spectrum. Some principles of adult learning suggested by Brookfield (1986) and discussed by Mulholland (1990) are also useful in considering how you might plan your education:

- Participation is voluntary. It is unlikely that people will learn well if they have to take part in an activity that they do not consider relevant.
- Provider and learner have respect for each other's worth. It is likely that an 'expert' lecture will lead to greater learning if both lecturer and participants are aware of the learning needs the lecture is meant to address.
- Co-operation between learner and provider should exist at all stages of the programme. It is not enough if there has been discussion about the content. The learning experience is likely to be more successful if there has been collaboration at all stages of the planning process.
- The experience must include time for reflection and analysis. A lecture is unlikely to lead GPs to change their practice unless there is time to reflect on the relevance of the material presented and to discuss how to implement it.
- The experience should foster a spirit of critical reflection. Thus it helps if a series of educational experiences are related to one another. There should be time at the beginning of each session to consider what participants have learnt in the previous session in relation to their own practice.
- The process must nurture self-directed empowered adults. Perhaps the whole point of continuing education is to help GPs to evaluate their own practice. This evaluation leads to the understanding of future learning needs and to their appropriate fulfilment.

Let us try to put a bit of flesh on to this rather dry theory. Your learning is likely to be most relevant if it is grounded in your actual practice and tailored to you as a person and to your needs. These needs may be conscious—such needs are termed by Pitts (1994) as 'wants'—or unconscious. Thus you are likely to be motivated to learn something if you recognize there is a need to do so. For example, I was keen to attend a lecture on benign prostatic hypertrophy recently because I felt unable to answer many of the questions patients were asking me about possible treatments for the condition. There may be many other subjects that, to quote Pitts (1994): 'need to be learned but are not recognized as such. There may be many reasons for this, ranging from ignorance to rejection . . . The identification and elevation of needs into the conscious agenda therefore requires some form of educational strategy.' That strategy should be focused on reflecting on everyday work. It might include keeping a daily log of consultations, performing audits, analysing critical incidents or attending a Balint group. A Balint group (see below) is an example of a particularly powerful educational method, because it allows participants simultaneously to identify and to work on their 'needs'. Other ways of attempting to fulfil your identified learning needs might include (Burrows & Millard, 1996):

- Library and MEDLINE search.
- Reading books and journals.
- Audiovisual media.
- Visiting colleagues, educational attachments.
- Peer-group discussion.
- Collecting and analysing data.
- Developing protocols, formularies, etc.

So far, so good, but surely it is not that easy? If it was, GPs would be doing all these things all the time and there would be no need for chapters like this one exhorting people to take part. What are the difficulties? Neighbour (1992) proposes a hierarchy of 'educational imperatives', analogous to Maslow's (1968) hierarchy of human needs. Maslow expands the basic point that ability to take part in 'higher' activities depends on more fundamental needs being fulfilled. Thus the need for love and friendship might be addressed after attention is given to finding food and shelter. Having found love and friendship, it is some steps further on for somebody to gain sufficient self-confidence to start to realize their full potential. Neighbour's hierarchy refers to vocational training, but it can equally well apply to continuing professional development. Thus energies need first to be expended in settling into a practice and to familiarizing yourself with the 'systems'. You might then start tentatively suggesting some improvements to the way things run, but it may take a while to have the confidence and security to move your education forward in a more radical way.

One of the books that I have found most useful in running courses is called *Active Learning, a Trainer's Guide* (Baldwin & Williams, 1988; if you are interested in the process of learning, I urge you to read it, it's not difficult.) The authors propose a series of overlapping steps for running courses:

- Establishing and maintaining a climate 'which is reassuring and sincere, which taps and releases energy and which promotes openness and sensitivity to others'. This may not be familiar to those reared in the traditions of British medical schools!
- Support. This is fundamental to learning and development—indeed to survival. It is not really about reassurance but is much more active than that. Baldwin and Williams describe it as 'the promotion of a willingness to forget self in an atmosphere of encouragement and challenge'.
- Stepping. As applied to a course it 'involves a series of steps, each dependent on the previous one being completed, in an incremental development of challenge and support'.
- Challenge. 'The deepening of the quality of experience for the learners, moving into new areas of awareness, involving varying degrees of risk at different stages of a course.'
- Reflection. This is about 'the evaluation of what has taken place during the course and its relation to life outside the course'.

Clearly these ideas do not just apply to courses but are fundamental to professional development. You may well have gone through these steps in your relationship with your trainer. Just because you are about to move out of the relatively protected environment of the registrar year, there is no need at all to feel ashamed at looking for a relationship akin to that with your trainer which offers you support and challenge. With such a relationship (or relationships—a small group can be very useful in this regard) you are far more likely to be able to recognize and fulfil your learning needs, as well as feeling secure and supported. In many professions a more experienced practitioner is available as a mentor to support younger practitioners. Mentors are beginning to be introduced into general practice education (see below). We have found (Sackin *et al.*, 1997) that peers can fulfil a similar function and that the two-way nature of the relationship has considerable advantages.

Opportunities for education

The Postgraduate Education Allowance

Since 1990, continuing education for GPs has been dominated by the Postgraduate Education Allowance (PGEA). This rewards GPs for attending approved educational events, to the tune of over £2300 per year in 1998. For this it is necessary to attend 30 hours of education per year and at least one course in each of health promotion, disease management and service management. There appear to have been only three advantages of PGEA:

- Most GPs claim it. This is evidence that they are attending some form of education, however irrelevant it may be to their needs. This was not the case before 1990, when most GPs had no incentive to bother with postgraduate education.
- A number of providers are offering a good range of courses in all parts of the world.
- It has led to considerable debate about how educational events can be evaluated and (less successfully) accredited. This will be discussed further in the last section of the chapter.

The disadvantages of PGEA have been legion. Briefly:

- It was bitterly resented from the start, because the money for PGEA was deducted from the seniority allowance, which did not previously have to be 'earned'.
- It rewards attendance, not learning.
- It has led to a huge bureaucracy, which has hindered creativity and spontaneity in educational provision.
- It favours lectures, as most regions charge a flat rate per hour for approving activities for the PGEA. Hence activities with more GPs attending are cheaper for the participants.
- It is very difficult not to approve applications for PGEA, as providers can easily produce impressive course plans. Monitoring what actually happens is difficult and expensive to do on a large scale.
- PGEA is only available for principals, not assistants, locums or retainees.

It is likely that PGEA will soon be replaced by another system, but, even if that is already under way by the time you read this, the PGEA legacy will no doubt be with us for a little while yet. This does not by any means mean that all is doom and gloom. Most regions have now accepted the limitations of PGEA and have found ingenious ways of extending its range. In my own part of the country, for example, up to 12 hours per year of PGEA can be gained for following a personal learning plan with the help of a mentor or a co-tutor. The region does not charge for approving such arrangements.

The large number of available PGEA-approved courses means that a careful choice has to be made in order to get the most out of them. Most postgraduate centres try and put on a good range of courses and these are usually cheap. Many centres have subscription schemes, some of which cover whole regions. A few such schemes (such as that in Wessex) are even more sophisticated and do not restrict their activities to local courses.

Personal circumstances and preferences vary. Some of you will have great difficulty, perhaps because of family commitments, in attending courses too far from home. Others may prefer to 'get away from it all' and take time out to attend a residential course. PGEA-approved courses abroad have been much criticized, but many GPs find that the enjoyment of a relaxing week in an interesting part of the world with like-minded colleagues is genuinely conducive to learning. Education does not have to be a hard grind all the time!

Having convinced you of my liberal credentials, I should add a puritanical note. The frequently advertised 'refresher course', covering topics from back pain to heart transplants, may not be of great value. Such a mixed content will probably not fulfil the educational needs of anyone attending. Of course, many of the individual lectures may be interesting and entertaining, but how much learning really takes place is questionable. Also the 'hidden agenda' behind what seems to be a rerun of old-fashioned medical school teaching is some cause for concern.

Traditional education

Be that as it may, for many of us some, at least, of our continuing education is likely to be in the form of traditional lectures and refresher courses. You can find out about what is going on in a number of ways:

- Contact your local postgraduate centre. The manager and/or GP tutor will be delighted to help—and will usually be open to your suggestions for topics, etc.
- Your regional director of postgraduate general practice education (known as deans in some regions) will be a useful resource for regional courses.
- Your local faculty of the RCGP is likely to run some educational events, which are nearly always open to non-members.
- Yorkshire GP tutors have set up an Internet service for postgraduate general practice on http://www.cmeplus.co.uk. This gives you access to courses throughout the UK, which you can search for either by topic or by postgraduate centre.
- Many national courses and courses held abroad are advertised in the *British Medical Journal*, the *British Journal of General Practice* or the free weekly magazines.

Responding to learning needs

How do you choose which courses to attend? In practice, attendance will often be dictated by convenience and interest, but ideally learning needs should be an important factor in the equation. How learning needs might be derived from day-to-day work has been discussed earlier. A practical way of doing this is to keep a record of consultations or other daily events where you felt some unease, some feeling that you could have done better. A formula for doing this has been derived by Eve (1994). He proposes the concepts of PUNS (patients' unmet needs) and DENS (doctors' educational needs). Thus, when you recognize a patient's unmet need it may reflect an educational need for you, which can then be addressed. The concept can be extended to the whole practice (see below). Further details can be obtained from Dr Richard Eve at the Somerset Postgraduate Centre, Taunton and Somerset Hospital, Musgrove Park, Taunton TA1 5DA.

As indicated earlier, it's possible to learn from many areas of life, not just from what goes on in the workplace or on courses. Experience (of work or of life in general) is one thing. 'Learning from experience' may merely mean the repetition of bad habits. True learning from experience involves reflecting on the experience and considering how changes might usefully be made for the next time. This may involve more work but is ultimately so much more enriching. Portfolio-based learning (Royal College of General Practitioners, 1993) is a technique by which such personal learning can be carried out. 'Portfolio' is a term derived from the graphic arts and is a collection of evidence which demonstrates that personal learning needs have been fulfilled. A mentor (see Chapter 12, page 211) is virtually essential to help clarify educational needs, assist in formulating learning plans, facilitate the process of learning, provide support and validate the material presented in the portfolio. Many regions in the UK support this type of approach and approve it for the PGEA. A mentor can be particularly important in guiding learners through major changes to their working methods. For example, Launer and Lindsey (1997) describe how even highly motivated GPs attending their extended course based on family therapy principles 'habitually use interviewing techniques that are severely constrained by ideas from the dominant professional culture'. These doctors were aware, for example, that they would try and solve problems before understanding what their patients' problems were or that they could be too paternalistic. Changing these habits involves losing a considerable amount of security, as well as learning major new skills. It is hard enough for those who are aware of the advantages of change. For those who are unaware, it is obviously much more difficult, and a supportive and skilled mentor is all the more important.

Groups

Support in learning does not just have to be from one mentor. Many registrars miss the stimulus and camaraderie of their day-release course, once they have completed their training. Nowadays there are usually opportunities to continue in a small group offering support and education in a variable mix. Examples include:

- Young practitioner groups.
- Locum groups.
- Co-mentoring (or co-tutoring).
- Audit groups.
- Balint groups.

There is likely to be a young practitioner group near you.

These groups can be very useful for support and for helping doctors to make contacts in a new area. A few are also educational in nature, but this is usually peripheral to their main purpose. Non-principals have sometimes found that these groups do not fully meet their needs so other groups have sprung up, usually targeted particularly at locums. These groups are supportive, but in addition they aim to improve terms and conditions for locums and help to secure appointments for members. The exchange of ideas in such groups helps to increase confidence and to allow members to learn some of the skills that are needed for doctors working in different practices.

Working in a small group without a leader can lead to collusion. It is not always easy to stretch people that little bit which is necessary for them to move forward. In devising our co-tutoring scheme in East Anglia we have tried to avoid this problem by having a 2-day residential course, at which participants start to acquire some of the skills of helping a colleague and of being helped. Participants learn skills such as active listening, giving and receiving feedback and action planning. They are then equipped to begin a mutual mentoring arrangement with one or more colleagues. The larger group continues to meet periodically (with its facilitators) in order to compare notes and to develop new ideas. As time goes on, participants generally gain greater courage to disclose more of themselves, in the knowledge that they will be heard and encouraged to move forward by a supportive and trained colleague. For some people this approach has given them sufficient confidence and skill to make major changes to their lives and practices.

Our approach is just an example of how GPs can be helped to support and learn from each other. There may well be opportunities for you to engage in a similar process. Knowing that you have helped others to develop, as well as moving forward yourself, is an extraordinarily enriching experience. Boland (1991) feels that the whole community of GPs should be supportive, that we should all be our 'brother's keeper'. Boland has been highly successful at setting up small groups of GPs throughout Ireland. These groups are convened by GP tutors. Their basic aim is performance review. The Irish groups follow six steps (Boland, 1991; quoting the New Leeuwenhorst Group):

- Choose an area of performance.
- Look at what we do—directly or indirectly.
- Decide what we ought to do based on:
  individual knowledge and beliefs
  the consensus of the peer group
  the opinions of experts
  the findings of research.
- Reflect on the gap between the reality and the ideal and the barriers to change.
- Agree on action to achieve change and a timetable for it.
- Agree to review progress after an interval.

A small group following these principles and led by a trained leader is likely to be enjoyable, supportive and challenging and to lead to improved practice. If you are convinced, try and convene a group locally. So far these groups are surprisingly unpopular on this side of the Irish Sea.

In looking at small groups, examples have been given in roughly ascending order from support to 'work'. Nevertheless, I am convinced that a well-run group is supportive, whatever its actual agenda might be. So, if 'two things can be had for the price of one', why not pluck up the courage and aim for a group that is more than just friendly and sociable? Why not set up a performance review group or perhaps a Balint group? Balint originally set up his groups for 'training cum research'. As well as the participants needing to undergo the 'definite but limited change in personality' that Balint felt was essential if the doctors were to understand their patients properly, the groups were also designed to help increase understanding of the doctor–patient relationship. Nowadays some of Balint's ideas have already been incorporated into our 'culture' and attending a group is a less intense affair. One of the most satisfying aspects of today's groups is that they are great levellers. Exploring patients' real needs is difficult and challenging and not even the most senior among us has the 'right' answers. Doing this work, knowing that your colleagues will take your feelings as seriously as anyone else's, is highly supportive. Why not taste the Balint experience? The Balint Society holds a weekend every September in an Oxford College. For details contact the Hon. Secretary, Dr David Watt, Tollgate Health Centre, 220 Tollgate Road, London E6 4JS.

Higher professional education

For many years the RCGP, and others, have discussed the need for a period of further education before doctors become full principals. Because summative assessment has, intentionally or otherwise, put the acquisition of basic competence at the forefront of the registrar year, there is all the more reason for such 'higher' education later. Basic competence is essential, but there is far more to general practice than that. The principles on which higher professional education is based are exactly those that have been discussed in this chapter (and on which this book is largely based). However, there are a number of opportunities that cater for the particular needs of doctors who have just completed their registrar year. (A project has recently been completed (Joint Centre for Education in Medicine, 1998), funded by the Department of Health, to research those needs in detail and to recommend what educational resources are necessary to respond to them.) Four types of higher professional education, which may be relevant to your needs, will be mentioned here. More details are available in a recent book (Harrison & Van Zwanenberg, 1998):

- Associate schemes, rather like a 'senior registrar' year.
- Higher professional education courses.
- Masters degrees.
- Academic traineeships.

Associate schemes

These schemes are designed to cater for registrars wanting 'time out to recover from the pressures of curricular and examination driven study before committing themselves to partnerships' (Salmon & Savage, 1997). In the South London scheme described by Salmon and Savage, the associates are attached to two practices each for three or four sessions weekly. The scheme also greatly benefits the practices, as only those practices which are demonstrably under stress can apply for an associate. In the remaining sessions there is time for the associates to carry out a project or research and to meet in a peer group. The benefits to the associates and the practices appear to be considerable. Do read the details in Salmon and Savage's paper—I'm sure you'll be tempted to apply! Unfortunately, lack of funding precludes this type of scheme from being generally available. The one glimmer of hope on the horizon is that the Health Act passed just before the 1997 General Election makes it easier to extend the registrar year to 18 months. The extra 6 months could allow registrars to gain at least some of the benefits of an associate year.

Higher professional education courses

A number of these have been set up over the years. An example is a course in the Oxford region described by Baillon *et al.* (1993). They are usually extended courses consisting of day-release and/ or residential components and with participants expected to do 'homework' related to their work within their practice. They are generally designed for participants who are principals and are modelled very much on the lines that the RCGP has been advocating for many years. In effect they are an 'advanced' registrar year, allowing participants to focus in depth on areas of their work where they might wish to practise to a particularly high standard. Perhaps such courses are nowadays more suited to more established principals, as the stresses of practice in the early years (when many young doctors are not in any case working as principals), and at a time when family commitments are often most pressing, may preclude such an academic approach.

Masters degrees

These again may be more suited to established principals but, if they can find funding, some doctors fresh from their registrar year find it stimulating to combine part-time academic studies with flexible clinical work. With many of the newer universities offering Masters courses, it is likely that a growing number of young GPs will see them as a good foundation for a career in an academically orientated practice. This will be of great benefit to the GP educators of the future. Up to now, postgraduate GP education has been kept quite separate from the academic world of the university. Most Masters courses are multidisciplinary in nature and usually modular. Several use a variety of imaginative approaches. For example, those at the University of Derby and at Anglia Polytechnic University are run almost entirely through the Internet. The multidisciplinary approach is of huge potential benefit to GPs, whose traditional training and outlook are usually remarkably doctor-centred.

Academic traineeships

These are particularly relevant for those considering a career as an academic GP. The London Academic Training Scheme gives the opportunity for doctors at the end of vocational training to work for a year in an academic department of general practice for seven sessions a week, with the remaining time being spent in a practice. This gives a good taste of the research environment without any commitment to a long-term academic career. There are some similar schemes whereby the registrar year is extended to 2 years, with, in effect, the 'normal' registrar work spread half-time over the 2 years and academic work for the rest of the time. Some university departments offer a more 'in-depth' attachment. At Nottingham, for example, the young GPs are in effect (and in name) lecturers and the attachment is for 3 years, again with some time being spent in practices. The trainees' research is more closely supervised than it would be for a 'normal' lecturer and there is also some training in how to teach. By the end of the 3 years, the lecturers should be well on the way towards their doctorate. Of course, such experience would by no means be wasted for GPs who eventually decided not to pursue an academic career.

The practice as a learning environment

Having read this far, you might be forgiven for thinking that continuing professional development can only take place outside the practice in which you are working. Unfortunately, in some cases this is true. Some practices are so dysfunctional that the environment precludes any chance of worthwhile development. Hopefully, these practices are exceptional and the majority provide an atmosphere conducive to education. Indeed, it is hard to know where to draw the line between education and practice development. If a practice is to respond to change—without which there is no life—all its members have to be continually learning.

There are several advantages to education based within the practice:
- It is likely to be relevant to the needs of the practice.
- It is based on the actual work people are doing.
- It fosters the growth and development of the practice team as well as the individual members.

- It is likely to lead to tangible benefits to the practice (e.g. less stress, more income).
- There is immediate and easy access to it.

How can one foster a good educational environment in the practice?

1 *By holding regular educational meetings.* Some years ago, I offered some tips on how these might be run in order for participants to gain most from them (Sackin, 1990). My suggestions were mainly about getting the group process right. More recently, Sylvester (1995) came up with some recommendations based on his survey of over 100 practices in the former Northern region. He proposed that:

- Doctors need to develop shared learning agendas with the rest of the team.
- Practice learning activities need to be flexible as regards timing and participation by relevant team members.
- The potential of case discussions and consultation analysis for useful learning should be realized much more.
- Evaluation methods compatible with education in an informal small group setting need to be developed.

It seems that young GPs are in an excellent position to help put these ideas into practice. They are likely to have seen many of them work successfully in their training practices and on their release course.

2 *By participation in audit.* If there was one benefit from the 1991 NHS 'reforms', it was the formation of medical audit advisory groups (MAAGs). These groups have helped practices to start getting involved in audits and now, for many practice teams, audit is part of the fabric of the practice. The whole process of audit is really about education. The audit cycle is virtually identical to the aims for Boland's performance review groups mentioned earlier. Doing this work 'in house' has the added benefit that members of the practice team are learning and working together. Indeed, one of the most important things I have learnt in recent years is that even the tiniest change in practice procedures is likely to affect most practice members.

There are other forms of audit apart from that involving the traditional audit cycle. Arguably, examining any area of work with a view to improving performance could be called audit. Significant-event auditing (Pringle *et al.*, 1995) is particularly valuable. The temptation if something goes wrong is to attach blame or, if something goes particularly well, to take no notice. Significant-event auditing is designed to analyse such situations in a non-judgemental way. For things that went well, it allows the practice team not only to celebrate the success but also to learn why things happened as well as they did so that the elements of success can be developed for future occasions. Similarly, for things that went wrong, analysis allows the team to understand the problem and decide if the problem:

- Was just unfortunate (e.g. a myocardial infarction in a patient for whom all reasonable preventive measures had been offered).
- Requires further investigation by conventional audit (e.g. noticing that two IUCD follow-ups and FP1001 claims had been missed).
- Requires immediate changes to practice systems (e.g. a patient asking for an appointment for emergency contraception on a Friday and being given the appointment for the following Monday).

3 *By working on projects together.* For example, many practices have recently been developing formularies. There is obviously a lot of learning involved in such a project and it is a bonus that the end-product is also of considerable use to the practice.

4 *By holding away days, etc.* Perhaps these are a bit less fashionable than they were a few years ago. A day or weekend working intensively together, probably led by an outside facilitator, can make an enormous difference to the cohesion of the team. It helps members to understand their strengths and weaknesses and how they can contribute better to the overall performance of the practice.

5 *By feeding back educational ideas from outside the practice.* Very often, when attending a course we keep what we have learnt to ourselves. Sometimes this may be entirely appropriate, particularly when the learning has been based on personal learning needs. Mostly, though, it can be very valuable to share the ideas with the practice. I know of one practice where, whenever possible, two partners go to an educational event and then report back to the others. This allows for a more balanced view of what happened and what was learnt can be made available to their colleagues. In this way, the benefits of learning on courses can be made so much greater. Not only will the practice benefit from the new ideas brought back from the course but also those who attended will have a chance to reflect on what they have learnt and to have it subjected to discussion and criticism.

Accreditation of education

At the moment, the only accreditation of GP education is by means of the PGEA. This means that GPs who attend enough education get a payment. It says nothing about what they have learnt or what they are like as doctors. Conversely, those who do not qualify for the PGEA may not be 'worse' doctors than those who do. Indeed, they may sometimes be participating in more relevant education than that which is approved for the PGEA. For example, a doctor who spent a year having some personal psychotherapy might arguably be more sensitive as a GP than a colleague who got his or her full PGEA by attending a week's traditional refresher course. Does this matter?

The present system certainly has advantages:
- Continuing education is voluntary for GPs.
- The system is cheap, as the PGEA was part of the 'pool' of GP remuneration anyway.
- The administration is relatively straightforward.

Advocates of a change would argue that this is not good enough and that the present system:
- Rewards attendance, not learning.
- Allows GPs to continue to practise without ever taking part in continuing education.
- Allows courses to be approved whose content is not necessarily relevant to the care of patients in general practice.
- Does not link accreditation with performance as a GP.
- Offers no reward for following an appropriate learning plan.
- Gives no accreditation for non-principals.

The challenge is to introduce a new system which responds to these criticisms but which is acceptable to most GPs and is not too expensive to introduce. Stanley and Al-Shehri (1993) have made some progress towards developing solutions. They argue that we are still a long way from being able to define, and therefore assess, the competence of a GP. For the time being, therefore:

> we must use the individual as his or her reference standard and seek progress from assessment to assessment. This approach liberates us from many of the threats implicit in re-accreditation and substitutes instead an ongoing process which aims to raise the quality of primary care through the professional development of GPs at a rate appropriate to the needs of the individual.

Stanley and Al-Shehri go on to suggest that such an assessment would be based on the doctor's ability to learn from experience, and it would become the 'formal assessment arm of this natural learning cycle for established GPs'. In other words, their proposed accreditation scheme would be based not just on GPs taking part in appropriate self-directed learning programmes, but they would also have to demonstrate that learning had taken place.

In 1998 the Chief Medical Officer (Chief Medical Officer, 1998) published the report of a working group he had convened to examine the whole issue of continuing professional development for GPs. 'The principal recommendation is to integrate and improve the educational process through the Practice Professional Development Plan (PPDP)'. This would be 'based on the service development plans of the practice and identified educational need'. The proposals take into account the principles of practice-based education which I discussed above, with a particular emphasis on primary-care professionals learning together. It is proposed that the system of PPDPs should initially run in parallel with the existing PGEA arrangements. Thus, acceptance of a PPDP by the health authority would trigger payment of the PGEA to the principals in that practice.

The CMO's report was written before the publication of the New NHS White Paper late in 1997 (Secretary of State for Health, 1997). It is possible that PPDPs will need to relate to the role of Primary Care Groups in implementing clinical governance and local health improvement programmes. This could lead to a system of education being accredited only if it is shown to lead to improved standards of care for patients—arguably one stage further on from Stanley and Al-Shehri's proposals.

If there are the beginnings of a more relevant system of educational accreditation for principals, the position is quite unclear for non-principals whose performance may be particularly difficult to judge. Berrington *et al.* (1996) have suggested that a modular form of education may be appropriate, with credits given towards future accreditation or further education, such as a higher degree.

Fellowship of the RCGP by Assessment

This chapter ends with a brief discussion of Fellowship by Assessment (FBA). I hope that you will see active College membership as an important part of your professional development. However, the purpose in discussing FBA is not primarily to advertise the College but to suggest that the process of preparing for, and achieving, the FBA encapsulates most of the good educational ideas that have been advocated in this chapter. These include:

- Learning based on the needs of the individual GP and his or her practice.
- The content and methods continually being revised.
- Input from the candidates (learners) into the whole process.
- Outcome demonstrably related to a high standard of care for patients.
- The need to involve the whole practice in the educational process.
- A tangible reward based both on effort and performance.

The aim of FBA is to reward College members who are able to demonstrate that they offer an exceptionally high standard of care to their patients. The criteria by which they are judged are absolute—no fudging is allowed—but these criteria are revised each year as a result of discussions with both assessors and candidates. It is virtually impossible to achieve FBA without following a detailed educational programme within the practice and preferably shared in a group with other candidates. The programme is based entirely on the learning needs of candidates, as assessed by the distance they need to travel from their present performance to that needed to meet the criteria. Candidates are strongly advised, when carrying out the educational programme, to be guided by a local adviser, who then acts as one of the three assessors. Here we have a successful example of a mentor who also acts as an assessor, a model that will almost certainly become much more widespread in general practice education.

Even if you do not intend to offer yourself for the FBA, I recommend that you use the criteria to guide you in your educational endeavours. Further details are available from the Administrative Office, Vale of Trent Faculty, RCGP, Department of General Practice, The Medical School, Queen's Medical Centre, Nottingham NG7 2UH.

Conclusions

Congratulations on reading this far—or maybe you are one of those readers who starts reading a book at the end. Either way I hope that reading this chapter has been as enjoyable and stimulating for you as writing it has been for me. Hopefully, the content of this chapter will have gone a little way towards encouraging you to be involved in GP education beyond your time as a registrar, not only as an enthusiastic consumer but also as an innovator and developer. That is the way that general practice will continue to serve the needs of our patients in the most rewarding way for the doctors.

References

Baillon, B., Flew, R., Hasler, J., Huins, T. & Toby, J. (1993) Higher training for general practice in the Oxford region. *Postgraduate Education for General Practice* **4**, 29–36.

Baldwin, J. & Williams, H. (1988) *Active Learning, a Trainer's Guide.* Blackwell Education, Oxford.

Berrington, B., Hibble, A. & Sackin, P. (1996) Higher professional education for general practice. *Education for General Practice* **7**, 187–190.

Boland, M. (1991) My brother's keeper. *British Journal of General Practice* **41**, 295–300.

Brookfield, S. (1986) *Understanding and Facilitating Adult Learning.* Open University Press, Milton Keynes.

Burrows, P. & Millard, L. (1996) Personal learning in general practice. *Education for General Practice* **7**, 300–305.

Chief Medical Officer (1998) *A Review of Continuing Professional Development in General Practice*. Department of Health, Leeds.

Eve, R. (1994) *Meeting Educational Needs in General Practice—Learning with PUNs and DENs*.

Harrison, J. & Van Zwanenberg, T. (1998) *GP Tomorrow*. Radcliffe Medical Press, Abingdon, UK.

Joint Centre for Education in Medicine (1998) *An Evaluation of Educational Needs and Provision for Doctors Within Three Years of Completion of Vocational Training for General Practice*. Joint Centre for Education in Medicine, London.

Launer, J. & Lindsey, C. (1997) Training for systemic general practice: a new approach from the Tavistock Clinic. *British Journal of General Practice* **47**, 453–456.

Maslow, A. (1968) *Towards a Psychology of Being*. Van Nostrand, New York.

Mulholland, L. (1990) Continuing medical education. Is there a crisis? *Postgraduate Education for General Practice* **1**, 69–72.

Neighbour, R. (1992) *The Inner Apprentice*. Kluwer, Lancaster.

Pitts, J. (1994) Audience involvement in a general practice 'refresher course'—the sharing of 'wants' and 'needs'. *Education for General Practice* **5**, 190–198.

Pringle, M., Bradley, C., Carmichael, C., Wallis, H. & Moore, A. (1995) *Significant Event Auditing. A Study of the Feasibility and Potential of Case-based Auditing in Primary Care*. Occasional Paper no. 70. RCGP, London.

Royal College of General Practitioners (1993) *Portfolio-based Learning in General Practice*. Occasional Paper no. 63. RCGP, London.

Sackin, P. (1990) Practice-based continuing medical education. *Postgraduate Education for General Practice* **1**, 2–4.

Sackin, P., Barnett, M., Eastaugh, A. & Paxton, P. (1997) Peer-supported learning. *British Journal of General Practice* **47**, 67–68.

Salmon, E. & Savage, S. (1997) A professional development year in general practice—the vocationally trained associates scheme. *Education for General Practice* **8**, 112–120.

Secretary of State for Health (1997) *The New NHS—Modern, Dependable*. Department of Health, London.

Stanley, I. & Al-Shehri, A. (1993) Reaccreditation: the why, what and how questions. *British Journal of General Practice* **43**, 524–529.

Sylvester, S. (1995) Practice based education in the northern region of England. *Education for General Practice* **6**, 118–123.

Appendix 1
Directors and Deans of postgraduate GP education (Regional Advisers)

The office of the Joint Committee on Postgraduate Training for General Practice (JCPTGP) is found at 14 Princes Gate, Hyde Park, London SW7 1PU.

Northern

Professor T. van Zwanenberg FRCGP
Director of Postgraduate GP Education, Division of General Practice, 10–12 Framlington Place, The University, Newcastle NE2 4AB. Telephone: (0191) 222 7028   Fax: (0191) 221 1049

Yorkshire

Dr J. Bahrami FRCOG FRCGP
Director of Postgraduate GP Education & Associate Dean, Department of Postgraduate Medical Education, Willow Terrace Road, University of Leeds, Leeds LS2 9JT. Telephone: (0113) 233 1517   Fax: (0113) 233 1530

Trent

Sheffield
Dr P. Lane FRCGP
Director of Postgraduate GP Education, Postgraduate Dean's Office, University of Sheffield School of Medicine, Beech Hill Road, Sheffield S10 2RX. Telephone: (0114) 271 2526   Fax: (0114) 276 8490

Nottingham
Post to be filled February 1999
Regional Postgraduate Office, Medical School, Queen's Medical Centre, Nottingham NG7 2UH. Telephone: (0115) 970 9377 (DL)   Fax: (0115) 970 9922

Leicester

Dr D. Sowden FRCGP

Director of GP Postgraduate Education, GP Postgraduate Education Department, Leicester General Hospital, Gwendolen Road, Leicester LE5 4PW. Telephone: (0116) 258 8119   Fax: (0116) 273 0296

East Anglia

Dr A. Hibble FRCGP

Acting Director of Postgraduate GP Education, PO Box 650, Anglia & Oxford, Central Block, Fulbourn Hospital, Cambridge CB1 5RB. Telephone: (01223) 219122   Fax: (01223) 219123

North Thames

West

Professor P. Pietroni FRCGP MRCP

Dean of Postgraduate GP Education, Imperial College School of Medicine, Hammersmith Campus, Hammersmith Hospital, DuCane Road, London W12 0NN. Telephone: (0181) 383 2138   Fax: (0181) 383 2103

East

Dr N. Jackson FRCGP

Dean of Postgraduate GP Education, 33 Millman Street, London, WC1N 3EJ. Telephone: (0171) 692 3250/3321   Fax: (0171) 692 3259

South Thames

East

Dr A. Tavabie FRCGP

Dean of Postgraduate General Practice Education, 9th Floor, Capital House, 42 Western Street, London SE1 3QD. Telephone: (0171) 940 9100 Fax: (0171) 403 0281

West

Dr R.G. Hornung FRCGP

Dean of Postgraduate GP Education, Department of Postgraduate GP Education, 2 Stirling House, Stirling Road, Guildford GU2 5RF. Telephone: (01483) 579492   Fax: (01483) 302163

Wessex

Dr D.B. Percy FRCGP
Director of Postgraduate GP Education and Associate Dean (GP), Post-graduate Dean's Department, NHS Executive, South and West, Highcroft, Romsey Road, Winchester, Hants SO22 5DH. Telephone: (01962) 863511 Ext 845   Fax: (01962) 877211

Oxford

Dr N. Johnson FRCGP
Director of Postgraduate GP Education, Oxford PGMDE, The Triangle, Roosevelt Drive, Headington, Oxford OX3 7XP. Telephone:
(01865) 740664   Fax: (01865) 740641

South Western

Professor D.J. Pereira Gray OBE MA PRCGP
Director of Postgraduate GP Education, Institute of General Practice, School of Postgraduate Medicine and Health Sciences, Barrack Road, Exeter EX2 5DW. Telephone: (01392) 403001   Fax: (01392) 403001

Gloucester/Avon/Somerset

Dr R.C.W. Hughes FRCGP
Department of Postgraduate Medical Education, Academic Centre, Frenchay Hospital, Frenchay Park Road, Bristol BS16 1LE. Telephone:
(0117) 975 7045   Fax: (0117) 975 7060

Devon/Cornwall

Dr A. Lewis BSc MA FRCGP
Regional Advisers' Office, Institute of General Practice, School of Postgraduate Medicine and Health Sciences, Barrack Road, Exeter EX2 5DW. Telephone: (01392) 403023   Fax: (01392) 432223

West Midlands

Dr S. Field FRCGP
Director of Postgraduate GP Education, Postgraduate Medical & Dental Education, West Midlands NHS Executive, 27 Highfield Road, Edgbaston, Birmingham B15 3DP. Telephone: (0121) 456 5600
Fax: (0121) 455 6291

Mersey

Dr A.G. Mathie FRCGP
Director of Postgraduate GP Education, Postgraduate GP Office,
Hamilton House, 24 Pall Mall, Liverpool L3 6AL. Telephone:
(0151) 236 2637   Fax: (0151) 236 3122

North Western

Dr W.J.D. McKinlay FRCGP
Director of Postgraduate GP Education, Department of Postgraduate
Medical Studies, Gateway House, Piccadilly South, Manchester M60 7LP.
Telephone: (0161) 237 2104   Fax: (0161) 237 2108

Wales

Dr S.A. Smail FRCGP
Sub-Dean & Director of Postgraduate Education for General Practitioners,
Department of Postgraduate Studies, University of Wales College of
Medicine, Heath Park, Cardiff CF4 4XN. Telephone: (01222) 743059
Fax: (01222) 754966

Northern Ireland

Dr A. McKnight MD FRCGP
Director of Postgraduate GP Education, Northern Ireland Council for
Postgraduate Education, 5 Annadale Avenue, Belfast BT7 3JH. Telephone:
(01232) 492731   Fax: (01232) 642279

North Scotland

Dr H.I. McNamara FRCGP
Director of Postgraduate GP Education, North of Scotland Institute of
Postgraduate Medical Education, Raigmore Hospital, Inverness IV2 3UJ.
Telephone: (01463) 705201   Fax: (01463) 713454

North East Scotland

Dr M. Taylor FRCP FRCGP
Director of Postgraduate GP Education, Aberdeen Postgraduate Centre,
Medical School, Foresterhill, Aberdeen AB9 2ZD. Telephone:
(01224) 681818 Ext 53976   Fax: (01224) 840670

East Scotland

Dr D. Snadden FRCGP
Director of Postgraduate GP Education, Department of General
Practice, Tayside Centre for General Practice, Kirsty Semple Way,
Off Charleston Drive, Dundee DD2 4AD. Telephone: (01382) 632771
Fax: (01382) 665972

South East Scotland

Dr D. Blaney FRCGP
Director of Postgraduate GP Education, Lister Postgraduate Institute,
11 Hill Square, Edinburgh EH8 9DR. Telephone: (0131) 650 8085
Fax: (0131) 662 0580

West Scotland

Professor T.S. Murray MD FRCGP
Director of Postgraduate GP Education, West of Scotland Committee for
Postgraduate Medical Education, 1 Horselethill Road, Glasgow G12 9LX.
Telephone: (0141) 339 8855 Ext 5276/4738   Fax: (0141) 330 4737

Army

Brigadier M.D. Conroy FRCGP
Director Army General Practice, Ministry of Defence, Room 50a,
Building 21, Keogh Barracks, Ash Vale, Aldershot, Hants GU12 5RR.
Telephone: (01252) 324431 Ext 5289   Fax: (01252) 340348

Royal Air Force

Wing Commander I.G. Cromarty MSc MRCGP
Head of Postgraduate GP Education (RAF), Department of General
Practice, RAF Institute of Health Education, RAF Halton, Aylesbury,
Bucks HP22 5PG. Telephone: (01296) 623535 Ext 7652
Fax: (01296) 623535 Ext 7599

Royal Navy

Surgeon Commander N.S. Bevan LRCP MRCGP MRCS
Adviser in General Practice, Fleet Health Office, 18 South Terrace,
HM Naval Base, Portsmouth PO1 3NB. Telephone: (01705) 725204
Fax: (01705) 725482

Index

Page numbers in *italic* refer to illustrations, those in **bold** refer to tables

abstract, critical appraisal 225–6
academic traineeships 266
access to care 236
accreditation of GP education 269–70
accuracy of measuring instrument 227
active listening 68
activist learning style 58
acute illness, general practice syllabus 41
administrative issues 178–9
    see also small business management
adult learning 5, 23, 83–5
    educational contracts 199
    educational triangle model 84–5
    mentors 211
    principles 84, 254–7
    trainer's role 197–9, *200*
    tutorial sessions 61–3, 65
agency staff 187
allowances *see* fees and allowances
annual practice report 183, *183*, 193
appointment system 44–5, 216
    improvement 246–50
        changes 249–50
        consulting style differences 248–9
        demand assessment 247
        feedback cycle 250
        GP response to change 248
        non-urgent appointments 249
        peaks and troughs 247–8
        success criteria 249
    RCGP Fellowship by Assessment
        criteria 246–7
appropriateness of care 245
assessment diary 48
associate schemes 264–5
'at-risk' patient care 236–7
atrial fibrillation management audit
    108–9
attitudinal issues 209
audit 106–9, 162–77, **162**

advice 167
choice of topic 106, 107, 108
criteria 106, 107, 108, 166–7, 170
data analysis 175–6
data collection 168, 170, 175–6
data interpretation 107, 108
educational benefit 164
evidence-based practice 147
practical aspects 106
practice-based continuing education
    267–8
preparation/planning 107, 108, 168
problem identification 165, 167
problem-solving approach 164
proposals for change 107, 108–9, 167
prospective trainers' skills 215
rationale 163, 177
re-evaluation 167
stages 165–7
standards 166–7, 170
steps (audit cycle) 163–4, *163*, 167,
    168
summative assessment project 168–71
    marking schedule 106–7, 172
    written submission 169–71
time scales 176
worker-centred approach 164
audit cycle 163–4, *163*, 167, *168*, 267
audit groups 261
audit report format 169–71
    criteria and standards 170
    data analysis 170
    data collection 170
    discussion 170–1
    introduction 169
    references 171
    results 170
    summary 169
    title 169
availability of care 237
awaydays 268

Balint groups 256, 261, 263
Bandolier 125, 132

bias 226, 227
brainstorming 90
British Journal of General Practice 125, 132, 205, 260
British Medical Journal 125, 132, 260
British Standard BS5750 238
business plan *183*, 186–7
buzz groups 90

Calman (higher specialist) training 21
case analysis 89–90
case discussions 35–6, 267
case reports 148, 229, 232
case-control studies 148, 226
cash flow 183–4
    capital 184
    prescribing 185
    revenue 184
certification statements 19, 97, 204
change management 235
    necessity for change 238–9
    planning 243–4
    process versus outcome 242–3
    systematic approach 241
    see also continuous quality improvement
Charter Mark 238
chronic illness, general practice syllabus 41–2
clinical debates 231
clinical significance 229
clinical skills 49–50
    basic skills 50
    GP skills 50
closed questions 70, 113
cohort studies 148, 229
co-mentoring (co-tutoring) 261, 262
communication in course organization 80, 82
communication skills
    consultation 67–8, 76
    explanations 73–4
    small group experiences 88
complaints *192*, 193, 209–10
comprehensive employer's liability insurance 188
computers use 217
confidence intervals 228–9
confounding factors 228
confrontational registrars 209
CONSORT statement 227
consultation
    action taken 110, 113
    active listening 68–9, 110, 113

aims 66–7
analysis at educational meetings 267
closed questions 70, 113
computer use 217
critique sheet 77
effectiveness improvement 75–8
empathy 69–70
explanation 72–4
formative assessment 47–8
health promotion advice 75
hidden agendas 67–8
joint consultations 38–9
learning needs identification 260
MRCGP competencies 137, 138–9
negotiating skills 70–1
open questions 69
opening exchanges 68
patient involvement in management 70–2, 76
patient–doctor relationship 75, 76–7
patient's account, eliciting skills 67–70
persuasive strategies 71–2
role-play 89
simulated surgery for MRCGP examination 136, 137, 139–40
skills 66–78, 110, 113
summative assessment process 99
trainers' teaching style 34–7
understanding process and outcome 110, 113
use of time 74, 75
video recording *see* video
continuing education 220, 252–72
    accreditation 269–70
    hierarchy of educational imperatives 256
    opportunities 258–66
    practice-based 266–9
    rationale 253–4
continuous quality improvement 239–43
    aims 243
    appointment systems *see* appointment system, improvement
    daily work applications 240
    data management 243, 245
    feedback cycle 243, 244, 245–6
    improvement knowledge 239–40
    leadership 240
    motivation 244
    planning change 243–4
    priority improvement areas 244–5
    problems 241–3

professional knowledge 239
resources 244
success criteria 243
tools 240
contracts 196, 207
educational 30, 199
costs 235, 236
standards 237, 238
counselling 201–2, 208
teaching style 59, 199
course organizers discussion groups
87–8
critical appraisal 127, 157, 225–31
abstract 225–6
check-list 158
clinical debates 231
conclusions 229
confounding factors 228
introduction 225
journal clubs 230–1
measuring instrument 227
methodology 226–7
power of study 228
response assessment 227–8
results 227–9
review articles 230
short-cuts 230–1
statistical tests 228
teaching effectiveness 231
critical reading see reading research
papers
curriculum 90–2, 94
development 91
learning objectives 91–2
customer satisfaction 236
customer service concept 248
CV 10–12
content 11–12
covering letter 12–13
preparation 11
profile statement 12
style/layout 11

data analysis 170, 175–6
data collection 168, 170, 175–6
defining requirements 173–4
data management in quality
improvement 243, 245
day-release programme 16–17
see also half-day-release course
DENS (doctors' educational needs) 260
depth of care 236–7
diagnosis in multiple dimensions 36
didactic teaching style 59, 199

discussion groups see small group work
distance learning for trainers 215
drug companies information 221
Drugs and Therapeutics Bulletin 132

economic analyses 149
Education for General Practice 205
educational contract 30, 199
educational meetings 267
educational practice environment
266–9
educational supervisor 22
educational triangle 84–5
effectiveness of care 237
efficiency of care 237
electronic health records (EHR) 241
empathy 69–70, 75
employment legislation 188
equivalent experience 1–2, 17, 18
retrospective approval 18–19
ethical committee approval 171, 174
Evidence-based Medicine 126, 131, 132
evidence-based practice 143–60, 220,
222, 232
connotations for primary-care
practitioners 143–4
context-sensitive checklist 159–60
definitions 143, 145–6
framing answerable questions 155–6,
157
implementation 157, 158–9
information needs clarification
154–6, 155
information sources 149–54, **151**,
152–3
mathematical tools 145, 146
quality health care 236
relevance to primary care 156–7
relevant evidence 147–9
primary research 147–8
secondary research 148–9
experiential learning 198, *198*
explanation, consultation skills 72–4
extended matching questions
MRCGP examination 132
summative assessment written test 102

false-negative result (type II error) 227,
228
false-positive result 227
fees and allowances 8, 9, **180–1**, 185
assistance with claims 196–7
Fellowship by Assessment see Royal
College of General Practitioners

Financial Pulse 238
flexible (part-time) training 2–3
formative assessment 35, 37, 47–9, 200,
    201
  assessment diary 48
  consultations 47–8
  curriculum 90, 91
  formal assessments 48–9
  simulated surgeries 140
full-time training 2–3
fundholding 190–1
*Future General Practitioner, Learning and
    Teaching* 54

general practice recruitment 24
general practice syllabus 41–3
GP fundholding 190–1
GP registration 21
GP's role 24–5
guidelines 149

half-day-release course 81
  adult learning approach 84
  brainstorming 90
  buzz groups 90
  case analysis 89–90
  course content communication
    82–3
  group discussion 89, 90
  lectures 88
  role-play 89
  small group learning (discussion
    groups) 83, 85–8
  trainer support 207
Harvard style references 171
health promotion
  consultation skills 75
  general practice syllabus 42
health visitors 33
heuristic teaching style 59, 199
hierarchy of educational imperatives
    256
higher professional education 264–6
  academic traineeships 266
  associate schemes 264–5
  courses 265
  Masters degrees 265
hospital clinic attachments 50–1
hospital training 14–26
  Calman (higher specialist) training
    21
  co-ordination with general practice
    training 24

educational content enhancement
    22–3
  feedback 23
  future objectives 25–6
  historical aspects 14–15
  hospital post approval 18
  middle-year posts 18
  monitoring visits 19–20
  new deal 20–1
  regulations 17–19
  satisfaction levels 22
  short rotations 25
  short-list posts 17–18
  statement of competence and
    attendance (VTR2 form) 19
  training scheme structure 15–17
hospital working hours 20–1

income
  gross remuneration 186
  intended net remuneration 185, 186
  sources 179, **180–1**
incompetent registrars 207–8
independent contractor status 179,
    182–3
  advantages/disadvantges 182
Index Medicus 149
induction period 30
information sources 221
  evidence-based practice 149–54
  training practice resources 35, 36,
    217
inner practice team 31
inner-city practices 182
insurance 188, 197, 210
intended net remuneration 185, 186
Internet access 217
Investors in People 238

Johari window 54, 55
Joint Committee on Postgraduate
    Training for General Practice
    (JCPTGP) 81, 97, 204
  attributes required of trained GPs 97,
    98
  educational advisory committees 92
  GP registrar representation 92
  regulations 17–19
  trainer selection criteria 216, 218
  vocational training monitoring 213
  vocational training scheme guidelines
    92
journal clubs 230–1

journal reading 104–5, 256
   MRCGP preparation 125–6, 132, 133
   see also reading research papers

keywords, MEDLINE searching 150
King's Fund Quality Initiative 238
Knowledge Finder 150

learning cycle 61, 76, 198, *198*
learning diaries 63–4
learning evaluation 60
learning needs 255–6, 260–1
   assessment 33, 34
learning styles 6, 7, 57–8
   questionnaires 58–9
lectures 259–60
letter of complaint *192*
library resources 46–7, 56, 217
   cataloguing systems 56
lifestyle advice 75
listening skills 154
   active listening 68
   consultation 67, 68, 110, 113
   trainers 34–5
literature search 225–6, 256
locality commissioning 191, 192
locality of practice 5, 6
locum groups 261
log diary 22, 23, 63–4
   competence in practical procedures 114
   summative assessment 110, 113, 114

management aspects *see* small business management
Masters degrees 265
maternity-leave 193
measuring instrument, critical appraisal 227
Medeconomics 238
medical audit advisory groups (MAAGs) 167, 267
medical records 216–17, 241, 242, 245
MEDLINE 56, 57, 150–1, 154, 217, 256
   access software 150
   searching 150, **152–3**
mentors 211, 257
   portfolio-based learning 261
MeSH terms 150
meta-analyses 148–9
methodology, critical appraisal 226–7

middle-year posts 18
modified essay papers 49, 99
monitoring visits 19–20˙
MRCGP 116–17, 119–42
   blueprint domains 122, 123
   consulting skills video 136–40
   examination structure 120–1
   general preparation 124–5
   historical development 119
   modularization 119–20
   modules 121, 122, 123
   oral examination 140–2
      contexts 141
      preparation 142
      topic areas 141
   Paper 1 (written paper) 125–31
      examination technique 130–1
      knowledge of literature 125–6
      marking schedule constructs 129
      new question formats 131
      problem-solving topics 127–9
      written material evaluation 127
   Paper 2 (machine-marked paper) 131–6
      common terms 133
      examples of questions 134–5
      topic areas 133
   prospective trainers 214
   simulated surgery consultation 136, 137, 139–40
   syllabus 121–3
multiple choice (MCQ) test 49, 99, 100–5
   areas covered 100, 101
   MRCGP examination 131–2
   pass mark 102–3
   practical aspects 100
   preparation 103–5
   question structure 101–2
   results 103
multiprofessional learning 25–6

National Vocational Qualification (NVQ) in Training and Development 215
negligence 188, 197, 210
negotiating skills 70–1
new deal for junior doctors 20–1
New NHS, The 191
new trainers course 215
NHS finances 184
   capital money 184
   revenue money 184–5

observational studies 229
open questions 69
operational research 44, 45
organization of practice 178–9
outer practice team 31, 32
outreach clinics 51
OVID 150

part-time (flexible) training 2–3
partners/partnerships 187, 203
patient lists 39, 40
patient participation in care 245
    consultation skills 70–2, 76
    health responsibilities 70
    persuasive strategies 71–2
patient–doctor relationship 39, 75, 76–7
patient's account, eliciting skills 67–70
patient's agenda 67–8
patient's language 70
peer-group discussion 256, 257
peer-review system 230, 232
performance review groups 262–3
personal development 43
personal educational objectives 22, 23
pilot study 173, 227
portfolio-based learning 261
Postgraduate Education Allowance
    (PGEA) 214–15, 258–9, 269,
    270
postgraduate medical education 204–5,
    205
    Directors and Deans (Regional
        Advisers) 274–8
power of study 228
practice development plan 193
practice experience 29–51
    clinical skills 49–50
    contrasting practice attachments 51
    educational contract 30
    first week 29
    formative assessment 39, 47–9
    induction period 30
    inner team 31
    joint consultations 38–9
    learning content 40, 41–3
    learning needs assessment 33, 34, 83
    learning opportunities 29
    long-term relationships with patients
        39
    outer team 31, 32
    outside attachments 50–1
    patient lists 39, 40
    practice accommodation 29

practice systems investigation 43–5
    preparations 30
    sitting-in sessions 32
    teaching occasions 33–4
    teaching programme content 83
    teaching style 34–7
    timetable 30, 31
    worksheets 32, 33
practice library 46–7, 217
practice management see small business
    management
practice meetings 45, 178, 193
practice systems 235–50
    defect rates 241
    necessity for change 238–9
    quality improvement see continuous
        quality improvement
    training practice experience 43–5
    variations in performance 240–1
practice timetable 30, 31
practice worksheets 32, 33
Practitioner, The 125
pragmatic learning style 58
preregistration year 26
prescribed experience 1, 2, 17, 18
prescribing costs 185
preventive medicine, general practice
    syllabus 42
primary-care management 178–9
primary-care groups 191
primary-care guidelines 149
private sector staff 187–8
probability values 228
problem registrars 207, 208, 209
professional development, general
    practice syllabus 43
profile statement 11, 12
psychosocial problems, general practice
    syllabus 42
PUNS (patients' unmet needs) 260

qualitative data 175–6
    validity/reliability 176
quality
    assessment 236–7, 237
    improvement methods 235, 236
    see also continuous quality
        improvement
    standards 237–8
    see also King's Fund Quality
        Initiative, RCGP Quality
        Practice Award
    variations in performance 240–1

quantitative data 175
questionnaire studies 227

randomized controlled trial (RCT) 148,
    226–7
    double-blind 226–7, 229
    publication guidelines 227
    single-blind 226
rating scales 49
READER model 223, *224*, 229
reading, practice library resources 46–7
reading research papers 220–33, 256
    critical appraisal 225–31
    evaluation of evidence 222
    selection criteria 222, 223–5
    READER model 223, *224*
reassurance 73
recruitment methods 226
Red Book 178, 196
references for registrars 203
reflecting the question 35
reflection 255, 257, 260–1
    learning diaries 64
reflective learning style 58
refresher courses 259–60
regional general practice education sub-
        committee 213
    appointment of trainers 213
    selection procedures 217, 218
reliability of measurement 176
remedial training practice 208
repeatability/reproducibility of test
        227
research 171–5, 176–7
    aims 172–3
    data analysis 175–6
    data collection 175–6
        defining requirements 173–4
    definitions 171
    ethical committee approval 171, 174
    interventions 174
    pilot project 173
    project plan 174
    study design 173
    study population 173
    time scales 176
    variables 174
    writing up project 175
research papers format 225
results, critical appraisal 227–9
review articles 148, 225–6, 230
role modelling 200, 214
role-play 89

Royal College of General Practitioners
    (RCGP) 14
    educational objectives 23
    Fellowship by Assessment (FBA) 238,
        246, 271–2
    GP registrar observers 92
    hospital training standards criteria 20
    Quality Practice Award 238

salary 197
sample populations 173, 226
sampling bias 226
self-awareness development 54
self-constructed training programme
        7–8
    day-release programme 16, 17
    hospital training 18–19
    short-list posts 18
sensitivity of measuring instrument 176,
        227
short-list posts 17–18
sick leave 208, 209
significant event analysis 107, 268
simulated surgeries 140
    for MRCGP examination 136, 137,
        139–40
sitting-in sessions 32
Silver Platter 150
small business management 178–93
    business plan 186–7
    cash flow 183–4
        health authority reimbursements
            185
        NHS finances 184–5
    checklist 193
    general practice syllabus 43
    GP's role 178–9, 183
        commissioner of services 190–2
        employer 187–9
        poor performance at work 188–9,
            189
    strategic planning 186–7
small group work 83, 85–8
    audit 164
    continuing education 261–3
    group development 84–5
    group facilitators 88, 89
    MRCGP preparation 125, 126
    'ownership' of group 87
    practice educational meetings 267
    storming phase 87, 88
    teaching methods 89–90
Socratic teaching style 59, 199

specificity of measuring instrument 176,
227
staff appointments 193
staff employment 187–8
statistical significance 228, 229
statistical tests 175, 176, 228
interpretation 127
strategic planning 186–7
stress 202
consultation skills 76
junior doctors 21
structured abstract 225
study design 173, 229
summative assessment 15, 23, 48–9,
96–117
attributes of programme 98
components 99, 100
criteria for competence 99
curriculum 90
historical development 96–7
log diary 110, 113, 114
overall results 115
planning 116
records 63
relation to MRCGP examination
116–17
structured trainer's report 113–14
video 109–13, 115
written submission of practical work
(audit) 106–9, 115, 168–71
written test of knowledge (MCQ)
100–5
supervision 57, 197
surveys 148
systematic reviews 148, 149
MRCGP preparation 126

teaching styles 34–7, 198–9
tutorial sessions 59
theorist learning style 58
time management, consultation skills
74, 75
Todd Report 15
topical issues in MRCGP examination
124, 126, 131, 133
trainer 195–211
advocacy 202–3
approval 218–19
audit advice 167
certification statements 97
counselling 201–2
course organizer communication
82–3

educational contract 199
educational support 197–9, *200*
employment responsibilities 195–7
expected attributes 214–17
clinical experience 214–15
documentation tools 216
teaching ability 215–16
formative assessment 200, 201
line manager 205
MRCGP examination video review
137
part-time commitment 204
place in medical education hierarchy
204–5, *205*
problem registrars 207–10
reasons for training 210–11
references for registrars 203
registrar relationship 98, 201, 257
transition to colleague 203–4
research advice 174
role modelling 39, 200
roles 195, 196
selection procedure 217–18
summative assessment video review
112
supervision 57, 197
teaching style 34–7
vocational training scheme links
206–7
trainer selection teams 218
trainer's report 113–14
checklist of attributes 113, 114
trainers' workshops 205–6, 207, 208
prospective trainers' attendance
215–16
training evaluation 60
training grant 213
training practice 216–17
assessment visit 217–18
selection 8
standards 213–14
see also practice experience
training units 217
tutorial sessions 53–65
content 54
evaluation procedures 60
learning styles 57–9
preparation 53–4
registrar input 63
resources 56–7
self-directed learning 62
supervisory relationship 57
teaching styles 59

uncertainty 156–7
    consultation skills 73
Update 125

validity of measuring instrument 176,
    227
Vancouver style references 171
variations in performance 240–1
    common causes 242
    special causes 242
video for formative assessment 112
video for MRCGP examination 136–40
    consulting skill competencies 137,
        138–9
    logbook 137
    preparation 136
    trainer's review 137
video recording
    consultations 37–8
        prospective trainers 214
    half-day-release course group
        discussions 90
    technical requirements 109–10
video for summative assessment 109–13
    demonstration of competence 112
    log diary 110, 113
    marking system 110
    referral process 110–11, *111*
    review by trainer 112
    submission 111–12
    tapes that fail 113
vocational training 1–13, 80–94
    equivalent experience 1–2
    historical background 80–1
    prescribed experience 1, 2

schemes *see* vocational training
    scheme
self-constructed training programme
    7–8
standards 213–14
training practice selection 8, 9
Vocational Training Regulations 1, 4, 15
vocational training scheme 3–7, 16–17
    adult learning approach 83–5
    aims 91–2, 93
    content 83
    course organizer's role 82–3
    curriculum 5, 90–2, 94
    day-release programme 16–17, 81
    GP registrar representation 92
    learning models 4–5, 7
    locality 5, 6
    range of posts 4
    registrar-centred approach 4–5
    selection guidelines 5, 6–7, 10
    structure 4, 15, 81–2
    trainer's involvement 206–7
    workload 115
voluntary sector staff 187–8
VTR2 form 19

waiting times 244
WEB addresses 56
Working for Patients 190
writing research papers 220, 222, 231–2
    format 175
written submission of practical work *see*
    audit

young practitioner groups 261–2